Mad Mothers

A memoir of postpartum psychosis, abuse, and recovery

Lorna May Davies

Copyright © 2024 Lorna Davies

All rights reserved, including the right to reproduce this book, or portions thereof in any form. No part of this text may be reproduced, transmitted, downloaded, decompiled, reverse engineered, or stored, in any form or introduced into any information storage and retrieval system, in any form or by any means, whether electronic or mechanical without the express written permission of the author.

Some of the names in this book have been changed to protect the individuals concerned. All the facts, however, are painfully true.

ISBN: 978-1-916981-58-4

For my daughter and husband.

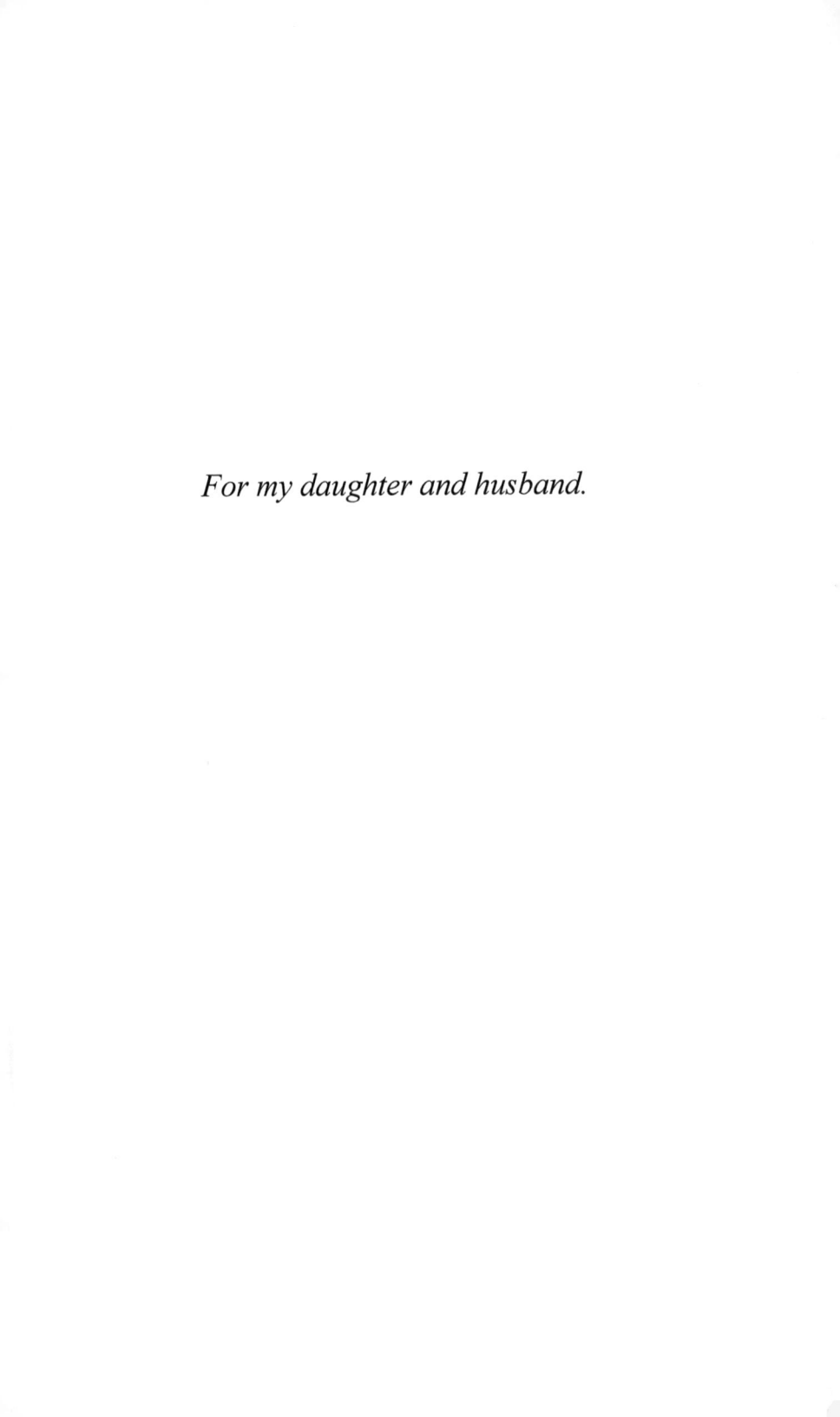

Contents

Chapter 1: How did I get here?.. 1
Chapter 2: My whole life seemed impossible....................... 12
Chapter 3: Big black cloud of catastrophe............................ 25
Chapter 4: I longed for some reassurance 35
Chapter 5: How would I manage? 44
Chapter 6: Dream crashed into nightmare............................ 51
Chapter 7: Danger to yourself and others 63
Chapter 8: Dangerous remedies.. 71
Chapter 9: I loved the MBU 95
Chapter 10: Recovery 106
Chapter 11: Trying for a baby 114
Chapter 12: A very bad joke... 131
Chapter 13: Incredibly unbelievable...................................... 142
Chapter 14: Senseless with grief 151
Chapter 15: Saying goodbye 159
Chapter 16: Walking with angels 168
Chapter 17: Dying 176
Chapter 18: A bloody nuisance 183
Chapter 19: Why had he attacked me? 191
Chapter 20: Left.. 194
Chapter 21: Domestic abuse 200
Chapter 22: A life worth living.. 215

Chapter 1

How did I get here?

The psychiatric hospital where I was confined didn't have bars on the windows but they could only be pushed up about ten centimetres so I couldn't throw myself out to kill myself. It was frustrating because I was desperate to die. Worse, I knew I had to kill my daughter too. It was the only way to save ourselves from the dangerous evil that was closing in on us. I felt frightened and confused. How did I get here? Why had this happened to me? Nothing made any sense.

The birth of my daughter, Natalie, was the best thing that had ever happened to me, but it was also the worst because it had caused me to go completely mad.

Once I brought Natalie home from the maternity hospital, I would stand by her white cot in our bedroom, next to our double bed, listening to her breathe, watching her tiny chest rise and fall, wondering how I should kill her. The voices in my head were insistent. They were just little snippets at first, half-snatched fragments of conversation such as you hear on entering a crowded room but then the voices grew louder, clearer and more demanding: they were talking to me, offering me a way out, a solution to all my problems. It was quite simple, the voices whispered, then stated, then shouted: "THE BABY MUST DIE" and "YOU MUST DIE." It was absolutely, incontrovertibly clear in my head that this was what I had to do: it was the only course of action. Everything else was very fuzzy and confused in my mind but this alone was certain and made complete sense. It was just a matter of doing it. I'd look at the white pillow on my bed and think how easy it would be just to press it down on her little face until she stopped breathing: she was so tiny it wouldn't take long or require much effort. I also became obsessed with the thought of drowning her in the bath. That would be very simple to do. "Never leave your baby alone in the bath," it states in the Health Education Authority manual *Birth to Five* given to all new mothers. I thought it was the most helpful advice in the whole book. I'd just tell everyone I'd gone to fetch a towel and, when I came back, there I'd found her, lying in the water, pale-skinned, floppy and glassy-eyed. Everybody would just assume I was in shock when I didn't appear upset...

I was delirious with joy when Natalie was born, even though she ripped me apart and I nearly bled to death. Yet, driving home from my parents' house a few months later, just Natalie and I in the car, I felt a sudden desperate urge to drive as fast as I could into the neighbouring brick wall, to end our lives, for sure. Both of us would be killed at the same time, which would be quite a neat solution. In all my other murderous scenarios I would kill her first and then I'd swallow all the paracetamol and antidepressants I'd been hoarding in my bedside drawer. They were still there: the blue and white packets bursting with promise. If I swallowed them all it would all be over. I was fighting the voices all the time, arguing with them in my own head, continuously. No wonder I was so tired of it all. I felt completely exhausted.

I also heard people laughing at me, constantly, every time I dared venture outdoors, pushing her in her green-checked pram. I'd taken to sneaking down back alleys now and hiding there, ashamed of how ugly my baby was (no wonder they laughed at her: skinny, sick-looking, red-haired little monster that she was) knowing that everyone who looked at me could see immediately that I was a bad mother, like I had it stamped on my forehead in indelible ink. Everyone could see at once that I was the worst person in the whole world. What sort of mother wants to kill her own baby? It is against everything that a mother is supposed to be. Mothers are meant to be kind, caring and nurturing, not psychotic, murderous, suicidal maniacs.

I was also seeing things that were not there. My hallucinations were triggered by the garish cards that everyone we knew sent us when Natalie was born. Graham had put them all up: on the piano; on the windowsill; on the table; on the cupboard; on the television. Everywhere I looked I saw cards depicting pink, smiling, baby bundles and they all proclaimed: "A baby girl, how lovely!" But it wasn't lovely at all. It was horrible because when I looked at them, the happy, beaming, dimply baby faces would change into laughing, evil, twisted faces and they would seem to spring out of the cards at me, devilishly mocking me, saying, "You've done it now, girl. Suffer and die!" I had to half-close my eyes to take all the cards down with trembling fingers. I wanted to burn them all and the whole house down with them. Whatever helped put an end to all the torment.

I was frightened of my baby. I feared myself. I was petrified of everything. When you go mad, the world becomes a terrifying place. Everything familiar is changed and becomes shocking.

Mad is so close to bad and that's how I thought of myself: mad and bad. I was a terrible mother I told everyone who would listen. It's all over my hospital notes: "I am a failure. I am a bad mother," I'm quoted saying repeatedly, an endless refrain. I felt I'd let everybody down completely and everyone could see it as soon as they glanced at me, I was convinced. Everybody could see me for what I was as they could read my mind; I told all the psychiatrists. And I always hoped and thought I'd be such a good mother, so that's why I found the fact that I wasn't so devastating. That's what had sustained me through ten prolonged years of trying desperately to conceive, through the hurt and pain of disappointment.

"When I do have a baby, I'll be a good mother," I'd told myself, over again. I'd vowed to myself growing up that I would never raise a child as I'd been raised: I'd do it right. And now I wasn't a good mother at all. I'd proved that to everyone and so I felt totally shattered. All my illusions about myself were completely wrong. I was the worst mother I could possibly be. How could I go on and why should I bother? All those ten interminable years of trying and suffering and living through the pain and torment of infertility had ended in a total nightmare. What I'd always wanted, what I thought I'd be good at, I was not. And there was nothing else. My whole life, my whole idea of myself, had been turned upside down.

Even now, I still feel guilty about how I was in the first months of her life. Has she been affected by that time? She must have been though there is no way I can ever measure it. I look at photographs of her as a baby and I don't recognise her at all. It's like looking at a stranger's child. In my mind I saw her as ugly, scrawny, sick-looking with bright red hair. She was always crying and vomiting up all the milk and food I gave her. Yet, in the photographs, she's lovely: a big, bonny, golden-haired, laughing little girl, bursting with good health. It is like I had a demon child that I can remember very well, who frightened and tormented me but, somehow, she was taken away by the psychiatric hospital and replaced by my real baby.

Some years ago, I found the courage, at last, to ask for my medical records from my psychiatric hospital. They sent them all very quickly, efficiently and without charge – a one-inch-thick sheath of closely detailed notes, checks, letters and observations. They thudded through my letter box and I read them on my knees in the hall, so frightened that my hands shook, and my heart galloped. It was a tearful, humbling experience to read through them, yet I was immensely grateful to have the means to piece together a time in my life I thought I'd lost. The notes fascinated and horrified me in a car-crash way. I couldn't stop reading them though they made me feel sick. There were many things I didn't remember at all, yet there it all is detailed in my notes, the same painful, embarrassing incidents as described by two or three different healthcare professionals. How I wet myself; how I kept laughing inappropriately to myself; how what I said didn't make any sense; how I was bizarre, having delusions, wandering around aimlessly, not able to do the simplest thing for myself; how I was confused, vague and distant; how I was extremely anxious and shaking all over. Other episodes I remember clearly, such as when I was told to leave a relaxation class for being too agitated and disruptive, are not mentioned in my notes at all. I told my husband Graham about the relaxation class fiasco and how ashamed I felt at the time, so he remembers it; but did it really happen? It's all very odd.

I doubt myself. I used to have an excellent memory; it helped me pass a lot of exams but now I question myself, constantly. I also check everything with other people. Nothing seems reliable anymore: this is what madness does to you. Everything is changed, forever: the way I see things; the way other people see me. Nothing is set and solid. Everything is wavering, fluid and fuzzy around the edges. It's a completely different way of seeing and experiencing the world. And I must learn to live with the stigma, the constantly present fear of telling other people or of acquaintances finding out.

Wondering whether I would slip into madness again used to be one of my biggest worries. People like me who have gone mad know how effortless it is, what a thin, easily crossed line there is between sanity and insanity, how simple it is just to step over and be gone, lost forever.

Now I know I won't go mad again, after all, I'll never have another child as I've been through the blessed menopause. That way madness lies. After I was discharged I was obliged to keep various appointments daily with a psychiatric nurse in my own home. I also had weekly and monthly appointments with psychiatrists and psychologists at the local clinic. I sat demurely in bland, clinical rooms with them, hands resting on my lap, trying to look relaxed while lying to nurse after nurse, psychiatrist after psychologist. All their questions led up to the main killer one: how would I feel about having another baby? The "right" answer, the one I learnt to give was: "Fine." The true answer, the one I learnt to keep to myself is, "I would perform an abortion upon myself with a rusty knife rather than have another child." I used to envy pregnant women so much, I could taste it in my mouth like green bile. Now, I pity them. You poor women, I think. You're about to go through hell itself. You'll lose your body, your own self and then your mind, as I did.

The worst thing about going mad was the fear of the condition itself and the stigma. All the time I was in psychiatric hospital, all the phrases about being crazy went round repeatedly in my head: enough to drive anyone insane in the first place. I felt I was back in the hectic school playground, children rushing around, pulling faces at me, making that whirling gesture at their temples, shrieking, "Loony!" There was not one pleasant way of saying it. All the euphemisms showed our fear of madness, our keeping ourselves at arm's length. But I couldn't distance myself from madness. I was in it and had to go through it and I didn't know if I would ever come out the other side again.

After my baby was born my decision to transfer to the public ward was, in retrospect, foolishly rash. I had torn very badly and needed the transfusion of three pints of blood and a whole medicine cabinets worth of medication. The private room I was offered would have given me much more of the rest I needed to recover. But my friend Julie had told me I would "pick up some good tips" off the other mothers, so I opted for the public ward instead. The only knowledge I rapidly gleaned was that I was a fool for breastfeeding. Every single one of the other women on my ward, young and old, every race, religion, colour and creed, were *all* bottle-feeding. They had their bottles delivered to them, all ready-made and together they fed their babies at the same time. They had contented, sleeping children and they themselves relaxed, gossiped and were very quickly into an easy routine. I, however, had no rest at all. My baby hardly slept, cried a lot and constantly wanted to be fed and cuddled. I envied the other women their leisure and peace. I was the only one who spent twenty-three out of every twenty-four hours with a baby stuck to my breasts. My child only ever seemed to doze for ten or fifteen minutes before waking up again, crying for her mother. Other people's attitudes didn't help either. I remember one afternoon I was breastfeeding on the ward as usual, and only one other mother, in the bed opposite, was present. A nurse came in, saw that I was breastfeeding and drew all the curtains of my bed around me, to conceal me, as if I was doing something disgusting. No doubt she meant well but it upset me.

'I felt like I was being treated as a pervert!' the woman opposite told me, when I finally emerged from the green curtains.

'Me too,' I agreed, sadly.

Later, a boy who looked about seven came to our ward to visit his mother, who was diagonally opposite. When he couldn't take his fascinated eyes off me feeding I felt uncomfortable, as if I was performing in a pornographic show. I longed for the nurse to come in and draw all the curtains around me then but, of course, nothing.

By Friday night-time I was physically depleted and emotionally spent. I sat in the gloomy ward for the third time that night, trying to satisfy the ravenous and demanding creature who was preying on me like a harpy, when, luckily for me, an experienced and sensible grey-haired nurse walked in and felt compassion for me. 'That baby is using you like a dummy,' she stated, boldly.

'Oh,' I said, not knowing what to say.

'Do you want me to take her into the nursery for the night, to give you a break?'

'Oh, please!' burst from me. I nearly cried, flooded with gratitude. I didn't even know there was such a place. (It says in my medical notes: "Help given to settle the baby," so this must be code for: "Took baby off to the nursery.") I felt like grovelling on my knees and whimpering, "Thank you, thank you so much." The kindly nurse who'd come up with the best solution merely smiled and wheeled the baby away in her Perspex cot, saying, 'I'll bring her back for feeding in the morning.'

Frankly, as I'd hardly slept for the forty-eight hours since I'd been in labour, I was so tired I didn't care if she *never* brought her back again. I plunged into my marshmallow soft and luxuriously comfortable bed and fell into the intense, comatose slumber of the utterly exhausted. It was the deepest, best sleep I've ever had.

I had to be physically shaken awake the next morning when my daughter was dumped on me to feed. I didn't feel happy to have her back. She came at me, her strong pink mouth open demanding, "Feed me! Feed me!" I felt she had the sharp beak of a ruffled chick in its nest, ready to peck. The baby was, as usual, famished. She sucked long and forcefully, biting my inflamed nipples between her bony, hard gums. That line of Lady Macbeth's sprang, unbidden, into my head: "I have given suck and know how tender 'tis, to love the babe that milks me." But only my sore nipples were tender: it was horrible. And it felt as if the baby was milking me of my very life's blood. She was like a tiny but deadly vampire, feeding on me incessantly, draining my essential fluid from all the veins in my body, sucking dry the blood from my vital organs, killing me, drop by merciless drop. But still I struggled on, trying to feed her. 'Breast is best,' I had been repeatedly told and like the good, obedient girl I had been brought up to be, I carried on, trying to do my motherly duty, not telling anyone about my strange, wicked, desperate thoughts or emotions. Surely I shouldn't be feeling like this? I asked myself, frequently. I had so wanted to have a baby of my own and had tried for so long. For ten years we suffered fertility treatment, enduring so much pain and failure along the way. But still I continued, still I had endured, knowing in my heart that I MUST HAVE A BABY and now, here *it* was, preying on me like an evil entity, an incubus, a devil-child! I was very worried, but I couldn't tell anyone.

On the Saturday I'd been in hospital three days and now it seemed it was time to go: all the other mothers on the ward seemed to depart after two or three days. Graham said his family were asking, "When is Lorna leaving?" But I didn't want to go home. I felt weak, exhausted and daunted. In retrospect, I really should have listened to my own doubts and stayed in hospital for longer, after all, none of the other mothers on my ward had experienced the traumatic birth that I'd had but I didn't trust my own judgement when it came to babies, or anything else. I had no self-esteem or confidence and I'd been brought up to keep quiet and be obedient. What did I know? Besides, I did long for my own comfortable bed, my own familiar house. Perhaps, when I was home, things would start going the way they should be? Surely in my own territory I would be able to love and cuddle my baby, and not be exhausted, frightened and anxious all the time? But it was a *big mistake*.

As I read through my medical records with halting breath and misty eyes, the hospital jargon made it all shamefully real. The notes were all about me, though of course Natalie is mentioned by name and Graham in passing as "the patient's partner" yet, what I most remember about being in hospital were the other people – the midwives, doctors, nurses, the other mothers on the ward and their visitors. There is no mention of any other patient at all: it's as if I had the whole hospital to myself, which is very odd. I was also amazed by the sheer number of notes written about me and the level of detail. I was only in for four days with Natalie and yet my records were over one inch thick. I was surprised by how much blood I lost (nearly four pints!) and the four long hours it took four separate doctors to stop my bleeding. My prenatal notes also made a tremendous fuss about finding anti-E antibodies in my blood. I didn't even know what these were and why everyone was so worried about them. They checked and re-tested me several times and finally concluded, "This antibody is unlikely to cause HDN or harm the baby." I remember being very anxious in my pregnancy generally, but I don't think I was worried about this as nobody made an issue of it to me. (Perhaps this was deliberate: all the healthcare professionals understood I was already extremely uneasy and so tried not to upset me further.)

They sent me copies of the consent forms I signed for my medical operations, one for the repair of vaginal and perineal tears, as I was haemorrhaging so badly after Natalie's birth.

The operation record for "suturing" (stitching two sides of a wound together) lists an incredible four doctors as working on me and the large tear in my vaginal wall. "Fat visible" it chillingly states and "persistent bleeding encountered. Mr. Yakabuski asked to attend 20-tennish." In ordinary language, they couldn't stop the bleeding and had to call out their top consultant to stop me bleeding to death. They flew him in by helicopter from his country estate, at great expense, a chatty midwife told me the next day. In only three days I seem to have nearly drained the entire NHS drugs bill for the year on my own, as I was given: Syntocinon (to induce labour);

Metronidazole (an antibiotic to prevent infection after childbirth); Cefuroxime (another antibiotic); Voltarol (a non-steroidal anti-inflammatory); Co-codamol (a codeine and paracetamol painkiller); morphine; Gelofusine; Lactulose (a laxative); Cefalexin (yet another antibiotic); Ferrous Sulphate (iron tablets); Erythromycin (yet another antibiotic) and three pints of blood.

It's horrible to read about the things that happened to me; the awful traumas I still have nightmares about, written down in chilly, clinical detail. I am flooded with upsetting memories of them, yet the reporting is so unemotional and full of medical shorthand. It's an appalling contrast. These episodes have scarred my life yet, to the medical staff, they were just another day at work. I'm not saying the workforce didn't care, I'm sure they did, though equally convinced that they must build barriers to shield themselves emotionally from the terrible things that happen to patients, or they would all break down. They dealt with my physical problems very well, but it was the mental fall-out from my ordeals that really caused me difficulties later.

The most useful thing about my medical records is that I can piece together exactly what happened to me and when. I went in on the Thursday and Natalie was born at five p.m. I can see that the only night I slept was on the Friday when they took the baby to the nursery. On Saturday night she is described as "demanding during the night." Is it any wonder that when I went home on the Sunday, I was completely exhausted, having had very little rest and been loaded with enough medication to submerge a battleship?

Once I was home I thought things would get better and start to become more "normal." How could I have possibly known things were about to get worse?

Chapter 2

My whole life seemed impossible

On Sunday Graham took us home. He had taken the trouble to wear the royal blue and black fleece I'd bought him for Christmas but his heroism stopped there. He did not know how to fit the new baby seat into our black Fiesta. He struggled with it for a while before giving up, leaving me to carry the baby in the back of the car, clutching her in a white-shawled bundle. I knew then symbolically, in that revelatory moment, that I was very much on my own: the baby was to be my problem, my burden, not his.

Graham radiated pride and happiness. He seemed so full of himself that I could hardly bear to look at him. I had no idea why he was so joyful. He started criticising me because I'd told him not to put his hand in my case. It was stuffed with blood-stained knickers and nightdresses that I didn't want anyone to touch or see, so badly blood-soaked that I knew it wouldn't wash out: they'd all have to be thrown away. He continued to nag at me on the way home and I felt like bawling. My eyes were glutted with tears, but I felt too tired to cry. I clasped the baby to me, but she was no comfort: she was the source of all the trouble. I felt so appallingly exhausted; I was on the verge of hallucinating. All I wanted to do was sleep, perhaps forever. The child had kept me awake for most of the previous night again, trying to feed incessantly. I knew I mustn't be feeding her correctly. Maybe the baby wasn't latched on properly to my breast, but they'd been so busy in the hospital that the midwife, who kept saying she was coming to check, had never been able to make it.

I longed for my bed like addicts crave an injection of heroin, but when we arrived home a jubilant Graham informed me all his family were coming round to see the baby as it was Mother's Day! I had no idea: I didn't even know it was a Sunday; I was so out of it. Graham gave me a card, purportedly from the baby, depicting a smiling, cherubic child and a blissfully laughing mother on the front: I felt sick. Only my Mum and Dad had come to the hospital to see the baby; now his whole family were coming. Graham seemed so pulsating with elation, achievement and satisfaction that I could only wonder: was he on drugs? I felt unbelievably low myself with fatigue and apprehension.

We had barely been home for five minutes when all of Graham's family arrived. My black hospital case was still sitting in our hall when they all trooped in: Graham's Mum and Dad; his sister, Janet; his nephew, Darren and his girlfriend, Kelly, her daughter, Karen. They were all so thrilled and delighted, talking loudly and animatedly that I felt like the only non-drinker at a drunken party. The baby lay in her blue-checked carrycot and had the longest sleep she'd had so far, slumbering blissfully through all the noisy chatting. For the first time ever, I wanted the child to be awake, to show her off to our visitors but, typically, she slept. I had a crazy urge to push her out of the way in the carrycot and lie down in it myself and go to sleep, I felt so shattered. My head was wilting with the most sluggish fatigue. My limbs ached with tiredness and felt as heavy as if they were made of mahogany. Nothing had prepared me for this incredible exhaustion. I felt like I'd run all around the world without stopping once. Why were all these people here? I thought, desperately. How long were they going to stay? Why couldn't they just leave me alone to sleep? And why were they all so joyful? I wasn't happy at all. I felt drained of all life and utterly miserable. I found it too gruelling even to smile at our guest's stories.

I longed to shout at them, "Go home and leave me in peace! Can't you see I'm totally shattered!" But obviously, I couldn't be so rude to my husband's family. They were normally lovely, and we got on well, but I was too exhausted to be bothered about anything. So, I sat politely on the brown sofa, sipping and not tasting my tea, making mind-numbingly banal small talk and pining for some rest and sleep. At last, after what seemed like several decades to me, the baby finally woke up crying and the visitors squealed with joy as they got to hold her and pass her around like she was the offertory plate in church. But nobody could stop the child crying and my heart plummeted. I knew it would be left to me. They all discussed, very loudly, what would stop her but only I knew what she wanted: what she always craved: my sore breasts in her tough biting gums. I carried the baby wearily upstairs to feed her in private, in her room. At least it finally got rid of the unwelcome, noisy visitors who were stopping me from sleeping but, unfortunately, they left me stuck with a child who was either crying or feeding for what was left of the afternoon and evening. Unless that demanding mouth was clamped to my breast, there were petrifying wails coming from it. I'm not criticising Graham's family. They must have thought, it's Sunday, it's Mother's Day, let's have a day out and go and see this marvellous new baby. They had no idea how dreadful I was feeling or how little I'd slept and nor did Graham, as I hadn't told anyone. I'd been trained to keep silent by my family since birth.

'What are we doing for tea?' Graham asked me later, when no meal had miraculously appeared, courtesy of the Tea Fairy. I just stared at him, blankly, the baby glued to my red, swollen breast, sucking away. What did tea matter to me? All my time now was spent in the same way: breastfeeding. Six p.m. was just like six a.m. to me: there was no difference at all. And how was I supposed to cook with a child cemented to my chest?

'I'll go to the chippy then,' he said, after a moment's hesitation in which I failed to bound to my feet and present him with a perfectly cooked meal from behind my back. Graham didn't know how to cook anything. I prepared the food, and he washed the dishes. That's how it had always been. I didn't usually mind but now, I just didn't have the time. This parasite was permanently stuck to my breast, sucking away, and I wondered if I would ever have time for anything ever again, even to go to the toilet. My whole life seemed impossible. How could I do anything with this limpet feeding away at my lifeblood like a leech: what was I going to do?

Graham returned from the Frying Tonight chip shop and emptied a few scraps out of the grey newspaper on to a plate for me. In truth I didn't feel hungry at all, which was so unusual for me, it had never happened before or since, even though I couldn't remember when I'd last eaten. I felt rather nauseous as I contemplated my future. What was to become of me? I had to eat and keep my energy levels up as the baby seemed intent on sucking all the strength out of me. I managed to stuff a few chips into my drooping mouth with one hand while cradling the child with the other. They tasted strange and grew intensely dry, sticking to my mouth like fuzzy cotton wool. I found them difficult to chew and swallow. All food tasted odd to me: I lost *fourteen pounds* in three weeks. I just wanted to sleep but the baby wouldn't let me.

The child finally tired and stopped sucking at about ten that night. I placed her in her carry cot, now situated next to our bed on my side, naturally, and tumbled into bed myself, stretched beyond exhaustion. I was too worn out to sleep and felt as if I was hallucinating, *feeling* my body levitating above the bed, sucked dry and shattered while my brain was twirling in overdrive. What was happening to me? Why couldn't I sleep when I felt more exhaustedly drained than I ever had in my life? How was I going to cope with this... creature? This wasn't the way it was supposed to be! All my baby books showed hundreds of photographs of happy mothers and contented babies, as did so many television advertisements and films. There must be something very wrong. My mind revolved over again, searching, desperate for the answer to my problems. Then the child woke up, crying, once more. Graham slept on by my side, snoring away and sluggishly oblivious.

I sighed, struggled into my dressing-gown and slippers, scooped the baby out of her carrycot and took her into her own white-painted room opposite ours, attempting to feed her. I switched on the electric heater and sat in the beech rocking-chair. She sucked me empty and kept on trying for more. The night stretched before me like a journey through a black hole in space. It was an infinite, endless void. The child suckled while the questions whirled around in my head. What was I going to do? Surely this wasn't right? What sort of life was I going to have? I needed to sleep. I'd barely slept since she was born last Thursday. Nobody could survive without rest, and I had all these other tasks to do; cooking meals; shopping for food; washing; ironing; cleaning; hoovering... and I couldn't do any of them because the baby wouldn't let me. I had a vision of my grey house crumbling into powdery dirt around me while I sat, child clamped to my bleeding, collapsed breast. And as for going back to work, that was just laughably impossible. How was I going to cope?

After what felt like several life spans, all of them wasted, pale light started to emerge behind the green curtains and filtered into the baby's room. Graham appeared in the doorway, naked except for his navy boxer shorts, crumpled and bleary-eyed, mumbling, 'How long have you been up?'

'Don't know, feels like all night.'

'You should have called me.'

'Why? There's no point. You can't breastfeed her. It's *me* she wants. Best if one of us gets some sleep.'

Eventually the baby did stop suckling and fell into an exhausted slumber but even then, I could not rest. I felt like I had been stretched too tight and might snap. I lurched around the house as my eyes leaked tears. Everywhere I looked I saw congratulatory cards mocking me and, inside, people had written how delighted they were for us: happy; blessed; joyous; wonderful; fantastic, were the words most often used. The pink, smiling pictures and messages all seemed to leap out at me and distort themselves grotesquely, laughing at me, making fun of me. I could hardly bear to look at them or be in the same room, so disturbing did I find them. They bore no relation at all to my experience: my baby didn't look bonny or smile; she looked like a pink-skinned rabbit who cried all the time insisting on being fed, demanding my milk, my time, my life blood. She had devoured me while in the womb like a cancerous tumour, leeching off me, growing bigger to become my Nemesis. I felt a sudden flash of hatred: I wanted to knock all the lying, taunting cards down flat off their superior perches and burn the lot.

The phone shrilled. I ran to answer it, pleading silently, 'Please don't wake the baby!' It was Stuart, Graham's colleague from the office. 'We just wanted to know how Graham was?' he asked, chuckling. In the background I could hear lots of other voices talking and they all laughed together at his words. It sounded like the whole of Stuart's office were all giggling at me and mocking. Graham had heard the phone, but he hadn't answered it. He appeared, lurking in the hallway, mouthing 'Who is it?' silently.

'It's Stuart, for you,' I answered.

'Tell him you can't find me,' whispered Graham, inexplicably.

'I, er, c-can't seem to find him,' I stammered, puzzled but obedient, feeling stupid.

The entire office all shrieked again, louder and more raucously this time, as if I'd told a joke. 'Why are you all laughing?' I asked, hurt and bewildered, feeling totally confused. I hadn't said anything funny, had I?

'Oh, it's nothing,' answered Stuart. 'See you then.' He rang off, leaving me staring at the black receiver in my hand, still hearing the mocking ridicule.

'They were laughing at me,' I told Graham, stunned, when I finally put the phone down. 'Why were they all taunting me?'

'I'm sure they weren't laughing at you.'

'Yes. They were. They were all jeering like mad. Why do you think they all laughed at me?' I felt really upset and perplexed, on the verge of tears yet again.

Graham took pity on me. 'They weren't mocking you. They were laughing at me.'

But they hadn't guffawed down the phone at him. I felt like I was going crazy. Nothing made sense. 'Why would they be giggling at you?'

'Oh, we had a discussion in the break the other day and I said, to wind them all up, that bringing up babies was just a simple matter of discipline and they all chortled away at that and said, 'You'll find out.' So, they phoned up just to laugh at me…'

'But they sniggered at ME… and it's not funny, not at all.' I felt really disturbed, tears prickling my eyes. After that, I constantly heard people chuckling at me as I laboured down the street, or behind me in my wake, as I left a shop. People sniggered and guffawed at me, continually, and would not stop. I had to hide up back alleys with the baby in her pram, so people didn't see us and chortle away endlessly. We had become laughing stocks, a universal joke.

But then the child woke up again, with that horribly demanding howl that I heard even when she was asleep. 'Is that the baby crying?' I always had to check with Graham, uncertain that I was physically hearing that wail I heard *all* the time. It vibrated in my ears and echoed round the house, never seeming to stop. Often, I was sure it really was the child yelling, and I would rush up the stairs, only to be surprised to find her sleeping peacefully. Her shriek tortured me.

'Yes,' answered Graham, simply. He wasn't tormented by it, that much was clear.

The doorbell jangled. A midwife stood at our door, to my astonishment. I hadn't known anyone would visit. Nobody had told me, I felt sure or maybe they had but my brain seemed to have stopped working. She found both the baby and I in tears. The child had been sucking at me continuously until I felt that I had no strength left. I was experiencing complete exhaustion and was becoming frightened of my own child and its constant, incessant demands. I was terrified of my own self, my black thoughts, my festering resentment and simmering violence. But, for once, I had some good luck. The midwife turned out to be helpful, my guardian angel in disguise. She was very experienced, took in the situation at once and was undoubtedly responsible for saving me from going completely under in those first few hellish days.

'The baby is hungry,' she told me simply, having listened to her cry. I was at the limit of my strength and patience, so snapped back, 'You don't need to tell me she's hungry! She always is. It's me she's been sucking on all night and all day.'

'Well, she's not satisfied.' The midwife fixed me with her clear blue gaze. 'You say she's not sleeping for long and spends the rest of the time trying to feed?'

'Yes.'

She sighed, leaning her head to one side. 'Do you really want to breastfeed? Of course, we always encourage mothers to, "Breast is best" and all that, but sometimes it can be really difficult.' She waited.

I stared at her, too shocked to answer. I had been repeatedly told, read and truly believed that breastfeeding was best for the baby. It was a mantra that had brainwashed me. But I had certainly found it to be true that breast was not necessarily best for baby's mother. 'But I do want to breastfeed. My mum did it for me...' I started to cry again, my tears spilling out. I truly felt like the most useless mother in the world! And I'd so happily imagined I would be a good, natural one.

My midwife made comforting noises and passed me a tissue. 'Well, from what you've told me about the birth, it sounded really traumatic, and you did lose over three pints of blood. That's probably why there's a problem with your milk...'

But I felt too tired to pay any attention to these wise, reassuring words. All I could think, or feel was *guilt,* the heavy weight of it pressing down on me. I was too incompetent as a mother even to be able to feed my own baby. I had failed and let her down; and she was only five days old. No wonder the child looked at me accusingly and then cried so resentfully. I'd had no right to bring her into the world at all if I couldn't even satisfy or look after her.

The midwife hung up her navy coat, said she was called Anita and asked if I had any bottles and a steriliser. Mindful that I would be going back to work and therefore could not breastfeed for very long (though the thought of returning to work was impossible at that point), we had bought six Avent bottles and a Mothercare steriliser. Anita showed us how to wash out the bottles with the new bottlebrush we had also presciently bought, sterilise them and make up bottled feeds with the Cow and Gate formula

Graham was sent to the chemist to buy. Anita stressed the importance of hygiene to me. 'Be very scrupulous about it,' she urged me, solemnly. 'Babies are very new, tiny and delicate. A tummy bug could be extremely serious indeed.' And this was the peculiarity of my mental state: when the midwife had been kindly giving me a valid reason why it wasn't my fault that I was unable to breastfeed, I had screened it all out and not paid any attention. 'Just an excuse!' I said to Graham, only listening to my own guilt. But, at this emphasised significance of cleanliness for the new child, my remorse seized on it and took it up, masochistically grasping this as a stick with which to thrash myself. It was as if, by this, I could make reparation. I couldn't breastfeed, okay, but I could make sure that I made the best bottle-feeds and satisfy my demanding child in this way. Both my baby and my guilt (they had chillingly become the same) would be assuaged. This was why and how I became so very obsessive about it. Even when others helped me, Graham or my mum, I would redo it all myself, behind their backs, emptying away the feeds they had made, rewashing the bottles, re-sterilising them, as if only I could do it properly.

Anita prepared and gave the baby her very first bottle and she guzzled the lot, like a ravenous reptile and then went right off to sleep, contented at last. I was amazed.

'When she takes three ounces well, up it to four, then up to five and so on,' the midwife advised, as she put on her coat to leave. When I looked at my watch I was shocked to find she had been with me for hours. 'Surely you have other mothers to visit?' I'd asked her, guiltily.

'They don't need me as much as you do,' she'd told me, truthfully, her candid blue eyes wide open like pansies.

Now she really was leaving, and I felt like screaming and grabbing her about the waist to stop her going, like I was a needy child myself. My angelic midwife had changed everything for the better, like a good fairy, with just the merest touch of her magic wand. Now she seemed to be reading my thoughts, as well.

'I will come again tomorrow to see how you are.'

She must have seen the desperation in my eyes and now I felt like crying with indebtedness. 'Would you? I'd be so grateful!'

'It's my job.' She permitted herself a quick, white-toothed smile.

'Thank you so much.' I saw her out, regretfully, still wanting to barricade the door and not let her leave me.

Now I had some new things to worry about, like hygiene. If the baby died of a stomach bug, which my saintly midwife had implied could happen, it would be totally my fault. So, I washed all the bottles and teats and rinsed them out and then did them all again, just to be sure. I rinsed the steriliser and bleached everything in the Milton fluid that Graham had also been instructed to buy at the chemist, scrubbing my entire kitchen with it and anything else the child might possibly put into her mouth. The acrid stench of the bleach permeated the whole house. In the past I had cleaned unenthusiastically but now I was consumed by it.

When I had finally finished, I stood by the baby's carrycot and listened to her breathe. I always did this now, terrified that she'd suddenly stop inhaling and exhaling and *die*. At least if I was there watching, I had the chance of resuscitating her.

Then our doorbell jangled again resonating through the house. I panicked. What fool was ringing our bell! They might wake the baby! I ran to answer it with Graham. We were both amazed to see a doctor there, as we hadn't called him out and knew it was nearly impossible to get one to make a home visit nowadays.

'It's standard practice to visit new mothers,' the doctor told us, breezily. (Why didn't I know this? I'm sure it wasn't mentioned once at all my antenatal classes.) We'd never met this doctor before. Graham absented himself, so that he could talk to and examine me.

Anita's parting advice had been, 'If you see the doctor tell him to give you water tablets to dry up your milk. Tell him, don't ask him, or he won't give them to you.' I, therefore, immediately asked for them.

The doctor fixed me with a cold look I read as plain disgust. 'Why don't you want to breastfeed?' he asked me. 'We always advise everybody that breast milk is best for baby's needs.'

I longed to explain that I wanted to breastfeed, but the child was always hungry and on my breast continuously as there was a problem with my milk. I wanted to tell him how I was exhausted as I'd hardly slept for days and just couldn't cope, but I felt too tired to justify myself to this demanding stranger, so I just found myself crying once again, the hot tears trickling disregarded down my face.

'I don't believe in water tablets,' he told me, as if they were Father Christmas or the Tooth Fairy. He continued, in a gentler tone, 'Your milk will dry up naturally once you stop feeding her yourself, but I will prescribe some antidepressants for you, to make you feel better.'

I brushed aside my tears with the back of my hand. I didn't want antidepressants. I wanted water tablets and to get some sleep. Why did people not listen to me, anymore? Had becoming a mother made me become dumb as well as invisible and sick? Yet, what else could I say but, 'Thank you.' Doctors always knew best, didn't they? I felt too feeble and ill to stand firm and get what I wanted. I'd been brought up to be passive and obedient: it's what I did best. I wished Graham was there, to back me up.

'When did you last open your bowels?' he asked me.

'I can't remember, doctor.' My toilet habits had become rather erratic as a direct consequence of childbirth and my irregular eating and drinking habits, I supposed. I had far too much to do and was much too anxious to eat but didn't have the energy to tell this to the doctor.

'I'll give you an enema to help you out,' he told me. 'Where can we go?'

I obediently led him into the downstairs toilet, feeling dazed. I was rather unsure as to what an enema was but consoled myself with the thought that he was a doctor and, therefore, he must know what he was doing. I was still bleeding heavily after my vaginal delivery and my surgery afterwards, and so was wearing knickers containing a blood-soaked sanitary towel, I was embarrassed to realise.

'Take down your pants,' he instructed me.

I did as I was told, *cringing,* my toes curling up inside my pink slippers. The doctor would see all my blood-stained mess! Why hadn't I flushed away my old sanitary pad and put on a fresh, clean one? But then, I hadn't had time and didn't know he was coming, anyway.

I hardly felt what he was doing. All my lower regions, indeed my whole body, had become an unfeeling mass that didn't belong to me since the baby's birth, as if the operation epidural had never really worn off. I just felt glad it was over so quickly.

The doctor had barely shut the door after himself when I suddenly felt that familiar, overpowering urge. I sat on the toilet for what seemed like an hour. All my insides felt churned up into a liquid mush and they just streamed out of me in a prodigious flood, while my stomach vibrated uncomfortably. Every time I thought it had finished, I had to go again. It was the worst diarrhoea I'd ever had. It went on and on…

Chapter 3

Big black cloud of catastrophe

'The doctor gave you an *enema*?' asked my life-saving midwife, incredulously, when she came the next day. 'That's hardly a sensible thing to do to a new mother.'

'And she's hardly been off the toilet since,' added Graham.

'It's true,' I admitted. 'I've got the most terrible diarrhoea I've ever had in my life... oh no... not again!' I groaned, making a dash for it. Thank god I'd put the baby on the bottle, I thought to myself, so that she'd slept for a few hours last night, satisfied, finally. The only thing worse than trying to breastfeed a child all night must be trying to feed a baby all night while simultaneously sitting on a toilet pouring with diarrhoea. My new hygiene obsession had been ravaged: already my hands were redly raw from over washing them before I touched the baby, her bottles or her toys.

Anita was upset on my behalf. 'You poor girl,' she sympathised, blue eyes shining, when I finally returned. 'As if you haven't been through enough.'

'It's probably my own stupid fault,' I told her, miserably. 'I can't seem to do anything right at the moment. I can't even seem to think properly.'

'I phoned the doctor's surgery,' Graham told Anita, 'to tell them about the diarrhoea, to see if they could give her anything to stop it and spoke to another doctor but he said nothing could be done. The enema would just have to take its course.'

'Not very helpful.'

Graham continued, 'So I asked the lady in the chemist what she should do, and she said to drink orange juice…'

'Orange juice? She sold you some, did she?'

Graham nodded, puzzled.

'I don't think it would help,' answered my midwife, gently. 'I think it'd make it worse…'

Graham's face sank as quickly as mine. 'Lorna's drank at least two litres since she got up this morning…'

'Well don't drink any more until it settles down. What else did the doctor give you?'

We led her into our brown-tiled kitchen, so she could view all my medicines, lined up behind the red kettle against the wall like prisoners about to be executed by firing-squad.

'Good grief!' The midwife gasped when she saw how many there were. 'You could open up your own chemist's shop with all of these. And why didn't he give you water tablets? I told you to TELL him, not ask.'

'I did. But he said he didn't believe in them.'

'Didn't believe in them? These male doctors! It's not him who has to put up with sore, leaking breasts.'

But then I had to run to the toilet, once again. It was my sore, leaking bottom that worried me at that moment, not my breasts.

'My breasts feel okay, at least, a lot better than the rest of my body,' I told her when I eventually managed to get off the toilet.

'Well, that's one blessing,' said Anita. 'Sounds like your milk was already drying up on its own, probably because of your birth trauma and blood loss. And another good thing is you've got your husband here. Some women are completely on their own.'

I shot a hasty look at Graham's oblivious face. I knew he would have to go back to work soon, as he'd only been allowed one week off. I was dreading being alone with the baby.

'Look at all these!' My midwife waved a dismissive hand in the direction of all the medicine bottles and boxes. 'Enough Lactulose to sink a ship.' A look of suspicion flitted across her open face. 'You haven't taken this, as well, have you?'

'Yes.'

'But it's a laxative!'

'Oh! I didn't know!' In between my dashes to the toilet, feeding the baby, obsessive cleaning, washing bottles, sterilising them and making up feeds for every four hours, I hadn't had time to read the leaflets on all my medication. 'I'm just taking what the doctor prescribed for me and what the hospital gave me. I don't know what half of them are.'

'I'll go through them all for you. Look and listen. Lactulose, a laxative: don't take any more. Co-codamol, strong painkillers to ease the discomfort of all your stitches: keep taking these. Iron tablets, to counteract your big blood loss: keep taking these. Paroxetine, antidepressants: keep taking these...' She went on, expertly sifting through my medication so that I listened avidly this time. I must have been told previously what all the drugs were, but I just couldn't remember. I'd been too traumatised and sleep-deprived to concentrate before but now I forced my foggy brain to pay attention. I took my marvellous midwife's experienced advice, stopped taking some of the medicine, kept taking the others and, after a few days, did start to feel physically better.

But after that first week, Graham really did have to return to work. I felt sick with terror at the thought of being all alone with the baby, and finally admitted it to Anita the next time she visited.

'Couldn't your mother come to stay? They often do,' she commented, her eyes glistening.

'She's already offered, thank god,' I told her. 'It was my dad's idea when I told them I was still having some diarrhoea. Dad says he and my younger brother, Richard, can cope without her, for a few days. They've borrowed a fold-away bed from my auntie and Mum's coming on Sunday night.'

'Thank goodness for that.' I echoed this in my heart. I knew I couldn't cope on my own. I felt bad asking for help, especially from my mum. As a child and teenager, I'd been the one to look after her. I'd been trained to do everything myself. I'd always been so organised and efficient in the past, as you must be when you're teaching; but not anymore. I really had to get back my equilibrium; after all, I was due back at work in July. Even the thought of teaching again filled me with shaky alarm. How could I possibly manage it? My biggest problem was, of course, the baby. She couldn't seem to keep her milk down at all. Every single day she brought back at least one of her feeds and not tiny amounts; this was not the usual meagre "posseting" written about so cosily in baby books; this was real vomiting, as she brought up foul-smelling, yellow, curdled milk in projectile spurts. I never knew when it would happen, so I hated feeding her because of it. I felt tense all over, like I was holding an undetonated missile. Then, suddenly, back all the milk would come, spewing out of the child's mouth like a geyser, drenching all of mine and the baby's clothes and all the carpets and furniture. It was like that scene from *The Exorcist* where the demon-possessed girl vomits green bile while her head revolves round on her shoulders. This was how I had come to view my baby: terrifying, bewitched, capable of unexpected, unspeakable horrors.

When the baby brought back all her milk as she did, at least once every day, everybody panicked especially me, as I was the only one doing the feeding. I tried to get other people to feed her, but nobody would. I got drenched with sick and got all the blame.

'You're obviously not winding her properly,' my dad told me decisively, the first time he saw the child regurgitate her feed. He was a father of the old-fashioned school who'd never fed, winded or changed a baby's nappy in his entire life and this was according to my mum, who did know. He was always at work when my mum was doing all this for me and my two brothers yet suddenly, he was an expert, much to the scorn of his wife. Typical of my dad, making critical comments, no help at all and typical of my mum: she had a go at my Dad; no help at all. His comments injured me profoundly, as usual. If I'd been well I could have overlooked his usual hurtful criticism, god knows I was used to it by now, but I felt so tired and vulnerable that I was immensely affected by every little thing. He must be right, I thought. I was guilty as usual: it was yet another illustration of what a completely useless mother I was. I couldn't breastfeed my own child and now I couldn't even bottle-feed her. I was so frightened that the baby wouldn't get enough food, wouldn't grow and would die; and it would be completely my fault.

Nor could I listen to the television news or flick through *The Observer*. Everything I heard or read I just knew was about me and the baby. All these harrowing things going on in the world were about to happen to me and my child: I knew it. A big black cloud of catastrophe hovered over us. But what could I do?

It was then I thought about putting the baby up for adoption. 'It would be much better that she should go to someone who would love and care for her properly,' I told Graham that night. I was desperate to be free of the crushing mountain of anxiety that the baby had brought into my life, not to mention the relentless menial work she entailed. I didn't enjoy her at all like all the "proper" mothers. My life was just one long series of endless daily chores: washing her bottles; sterilising them; making up feeds; the baby being sick; having to change her. This was an enormous and dreadful task, like trying to dress an octopus made of pink jelly in a string vest. The child wriggled so much and screamed and seemed to have far too many limbs to fit into the clothes. My sister-in-law, Janet, bought her a gorgeous pair of white lacy tights to wear under a red velvet dress. The frock itself was difficult enough to squeeze her into but the tights were simply impossible. How was I supposed to get her into them? Her legs didn't stop moving for one second. Then I had to change my own vomit-soaked clothes; remove the baby's reeking nappy and then, the horror of it, bathe her. This was the very worst in the whole catalogue of Terrible Things That Had to Be Done. The child truly loathed, with enormous passion, everything about being bathed. Having her sick-drenched clothes taken off; her face washed with tiny blobs of cotton wool; water splashed on her wisps of ginger hair to clean it; being held in the lukewarm liquid. She screamed throughout at the top of her bawling lungs, just as she'd screeched in the hospital when the midwife had first washed her, showing me what to do.

'Lots of babies don't like being bathed,' said the midwife, prosaically. (But I didn't hear any of the other babies yelling as loudly as mine.) 'She'll get used to it.' But she did NOT get used to it: if anything, she seemed to yell even louder each time I bathed her. The baby screamed as though she feared I was trying to murder her. How did she know? I thought. She must have sensed it: that tiny seed planted in my brain which soon sprouted and flowered and spread like poison ivy, threatening to take over every other thought in my mind.

Graham laughed about adoption, thinking I was joking. 'We couldn't possibly do that,' he said. He knew the child was a lot of work, but I'd soon get into a routine and bond properly with her. I was trapped but...

"Never leave a baby alone in the bath; they can drown in only a few inches of water," my baby book informed me, usefully, for once. Is that all it would take? I thought, trying

NOT to think of it, as I swished my hand about in the dangerous, lukewarm few inches. All I would need to do would be to go to the airing cupboard, to fetch a clean towel and, when I came back: disaster! There would be the child, bobbing face down in the water, blue-skinned, not breathing, *dead*. I could hear my voice telling the young policeman, "I only went to fetch a towel… to answer the phone… to get the door… I was only away for a minute. How did this happen?" But would he notice I wasn't crying and was strangely composed, that I viewed my baby's dead body with unusual equanimity? I was *free* now to live my own life, like all the mothers wished aloud for at the baby clinic: "I want my life back. I need to do something for ME," I'd heard them chant over and over again like a prayer, a special mantra, always that perpetual struggle between the two impulses: the old, selfish survival instinct that everyone had and needed to live their lives, warring with the new maternal urge, that strongest human bond a mother has with its young, the motive to nurture, to love and protect: NOT TO KILL. But it would be so easy. It would only take a few seconds. Of course, I stifled the inclination. I was an evil monster: I knew it. Who could even think of such a thing? It was against everything that being a mother was supposed to be. But however far I pushed these wicked thoughts down again, they stayed in my mind and grew, multiplying fast, poisoning everything in their inexorable path, like chemotherapy.

My day was one long, mind-numbing round of chores. One thankless, dull task after another to be repeated over and over again like housework, so time-consuming and useless. I'd never been good with boredom: I needed my mind stimulated. Was this monotonous robot all I had become? Why had I even wanted to be a mother? I had spent the last ten years of my life enduring all that painful, degrading, expensive fertility treatment; and for what? *This?* Why had nobody told me it was this bad? Why had nobody prepared me for how terrible it was? I'd looked after Richard, my brother who was eight years younger, when he was born but he'd been a good baby, no trouble at all, not like mine. I hadn't got involved with any of my friend's babies. I'd wanted a child myself and for so long that I felt it to be such an offensive catastrophe when my friends had a baby that I couldn't *bear* it. I would visit once, with an expensively wrapped present, leave as soon as I could and then break off all contact. I thought I'd know intuitively what to do, that my maternal instinct would take over and that I'd be a natural earth mother: but I just wasn't. I could not believe it. What was wrong with me and with my baby?

I was terrified of my own child and especially of my evil thoughts about her. I was exhausted by the ceaseless round of toil (most of it self-inflicted, it had to be said). I panicked when the baby cried. What did she want? I just didn't know what was amiss with her and this worried me endlessly. I was so horrified that something awful was going to happen. I had such a vivid sense of approaching catastrophe that it was almost like a presence in the room with me that I could see, touch and smell. I knew it was irrational, but I just couldn't help it. I told Graham that I held two completely opposing opinions. One, that nobody could look after my baby as well as I could (and surely all "normal" mums felt like this?), and two, the opposite view was just as strongly held by me: that ANYBODY could look after the child better than I could. I firmly believed both conflicting views very intensely indeed.

'But that doesn't make any sense,' the rational Graham told me. He might as well have been talking Aramaic for all the impact he made on me. *I* found it perfectly logical that I could think two entirely antithetical viewpoints simultaneously.

I felt so frightened of my baby. She was so unpredictable. Anything could happen with her at any time. I hadn't really expected to survive childbirth and I very nearly didn't, and part of my irrational mind had never assumed the baby would be born alive: I was convinced she'd be born *dead*. I hadn't really dared to think about what would happen once the child was born, as it seemed like tempting fate. Every single item I bought, very late, for the baby's arrival, I always wondered: would it ever be used? I looked at all the pink flowers and silly cards that people sent when the child was born, and thought: don't send flowers and cards, send practical help. I'm going under here. The nauseating cards all screamed forth: "A baby girl: how wonderful!" but I knew they were mocking me. It wasn't wonderful at all: it was terrible: I had made the greatest mistake of my life and there was no way I could get out of it.

I knew that I wasn't well enough to look after a child. I did not have the strength to cope. I felt so weak from my extensive loss of blood, my dearth of sleep and the gargantuan doses of antibiotics and antidepressants I was prescribed. I was sweating and shaking all the time, whether from my anxiety, my hormones, my medication or all three combined. I still felt feeble from the chronic diarrhoea caused by the enema the doctor gave me. I'd had less control over my bowels and needed nappies more than the baby. Now I'd developed cystitis and felt I'd lost control of my bladder too, and this made me feel even more insecure. And I felt so deeply anxious. I was always in a panic. Every little thing was a *crisis*. I lived my life lurching from one harrowing feed to another.

At night while Graham slept, tired and contented, I did not. I simply could not sleep. I stood by the baby's cot and listened to her breathe. I was absolutely terrified of cot death. What if she just stopped breathing? What would I do? I did not know. I stood watching and being attentive to her, night and day. I was exhausted, devoured by anxiety and hypervigilance.

Graham was worried about me, I could tell. I really wanted him there all the time but even in my highly irrational state, I knew this was impossible: one of us had to go to work and earn money to pay the bills and I couldn't, so he had to. He asked me what was troubling me specifically, so I told him, and he made helpful suggestions: Why didn't I make up all the feeds I needed for that day the night before, when he was there to mind the baby? Why didn't I make myself a tuna sandwich for my lunch, leaving it wrapped in a plastic bag in the fridge for when I needed it? And he would call for a takeaway on his way home, so I didn't have to worry about making our dinner. So, that way, he explained to me patiently, I only had to deal with the child: nothing else. I knew I was lucky and blessed to have my husband and baby. Why couldn't I just accept it? As Graham told me, philosophically, we had been trying for exactly this for the past ten years and I should be ENJOYING IT!

Only, I wasn't. I hated it. Graham was trying to help me, but it was like he was attempting to solve my illogical problems using logic. Despite his best intentions, nothing helped. *I hated* my life. I kept doing what everybody advised me to do, numbering my blessings and reminding myself how lucky I was. I had what every woman is supposed to want: a healthy baby; a husband who loved me; family; friends; a lovely house; a decent car; a good career; enough money. I knew I should be overjoyed with happiness but my foolish anxiety and lack of confidence with the child were crippling me. I was incredibly tired. Caring for myself came last of all on my "to do" list. I hardly had an instant to myself and, when I did, all I wanted to do was rest and sleep. I had never felt more exhausted. I was like a machine about to run out of fuel, and I knew it, feeling positive I would soon just collapse completely. Surely my life would soon slow down and become "normal" again. I just wanted to watch an episode of *Coronation Street* or read a few pages of *The Observer* on a Sunday: that wasn't too much to ask, was it? Surely the worst must be over, and I could reclaim my life? How wrong I was.

Chapter 4

I longed for some reassurance

It happened first thing one Monday morning after we'd both woken up. The baby was lying on her changing mat, skinny legs kicking away, when I found *blood*. I panicked badly. It seemed to be coming from her navel. Luckily it was the one morning of the week when an open surgery (meaning no appointment necessary) was in operation at my doctor's surgery, so I scooped up the baby, wrapped her in several pink layers against the April chill, strapped her in her pram and *ran* all the way to the doctor's, ignoring the turbulent dark clouds I could see massing above my head. I felt as if my heart might explode.

There were so many sick strangers before us we had to remain cooped up in the grim waiting room for over an hour to be seen. The baby was grouchy, unused to being in such a confined space and surrounded by unfamiliar people, but I worked maniacally at trying to keep her amused. By the time I got to see a doctor, I felt half-dead with anxiety and weariness. My nerves were tightened to snapping point. My hands shook as I unfastened the hundreds of press-studs on her pink romper suit and white buttoned down vest, to show the elderly doctor the bloodied navel. He reassured me, almost, that this sometimes happened: the child was not about to bleed to death, as I had feared. He gave me some medical wipes to clean it up. I was grovellingly grateful for the comfort of his words and dragged myself home again, exhausted and relieved. I collapsed on the brown couch with the baby on top of me.

Taking the baby to the doctor's for her check-ups and immunisation injections was just as harrowing, but at least I had prior warning that these were about to happen, as heralded in the sternly authoritarian appointment letters that descended, uninvited, through my letterbox. I would make my way to the doctor's surgery and up the stairs to the practice nurse's waiting room with lead in my guts. There were always other babies waiting for their injections and, to my jaundiced eye, they were always bigger, prettier, better-behaved and better-dressed, with much calmer better-organised mothers with them. There was one child I admired intensely belonging to a woman I'd met at my antenatal class at the local clinic. Trinny was one of those effortlessly exquisite blonde women who look even more radiant during pregnancy. Even at seven months, as she was when I first met her, she was still enviably slim, with only a tiny bump to attest to her expectant state but her peachy skin, golden hair and sapphire-blue eyes shone with a seemingly divine glow. She was also, amazingly, one of those friendly and engaging women that it's impossible to dislike, in spite of her awe-inspiring beauty. Her daughter, the aptly named Belle was perfection in baby form, with white-blonde curls, huge violet eyes and an ever-smiling, doll-like face. She dimpled and gurgled away on her mother's lap, like a baby from a Pampers advertisement on television. They both seemed so faultless; I could only gaze upon them with wonder.

I, of course, would get there late. I was already anxious and exhausted, feeling sick with trepidation, and my baby was uneasy and apprehensive, starting to snivel. I was weighed down with bottles of water, rattles, cuddly toys and blankets. I carried so much stuff around with me that everything got mixed up and pushed to the bottom of my huge bag, so, invariably, I could never find anything.

I regarded Trinny with total astonishment. She seemed to be one of those lucky have-it-all women I'd only read about in *Hello! Magazine*, who dance through life enjoying everything wonderful that happens to them, evading the bad things. Pregnancy had only added to the pleasure and joy in her already enviable life and her daughter, Belle, made it perfect. She was, naturally, one of those miraculous babies who sleep all through the night from the very start, breastfeed easily and for short periods, are *never* sick or cry. As Trinny and the other mothers recounted, unselfconsciously, their baby's marvellous habits, I felt myself tinge a most unbecomingly jealous shade of green. It didn't help that Trinny lived in the most desirable road in the whole neighbourhood in which all the houses were detached mansions with fabulous gardens and that she drove, very expertly, a midnight-blue, top-of-the-range Audi.

I could not help comparing my own rather ordinary lifestyle and troublesome daughter with Trinny's picture-perfect existence, which made me feel even more anxious and depressed. It was a relief when the charming and chatty Trinny took the stunning Belle in for her immunisation first. Surely her baby couldn't be as sublime as she made out? She *must* be exaggerating.

I asked my mum on the phone that night, angling for badly needed reassurance. I did not get it. 'Well, all three of you were very good babies who always slept through the night, breastfed easily, were hardly sick or cried…' My heart plummeted in despair. Surely my mum was looking back over the nearly forty years since she'd had her three children through rose-tinted glasses. I'd overlooked the fact, in my exhausted state, that she was Queen of Denial, and not in the Cleopatra sense. Either that or it really was, as usual, totally my own fault. I was obviously doing everything wrong, and I truly *deserved* to have The Baby from Hell, who didn't sleep, didn't feed and was sick and crying all the time.

Then it was my turn to take the child in to the nurse. My hands trembled as I popped open the endless press-studs on her romper suit, to expose her leg for the injection. Why hadn't I dressed the baby in her blue velvet dress that could just be flipped up to uncover her thigh, like Trinny had clothed Belle? My mind just didn't seem to be working anymore. Pregnancy and motherhood combined had destroyed all my brain cells. I was afraid I would vomit as I watched the point of the hypodermic needle being jabbed into my baby's unblemished, dewy pink skin. I would much rather have had it rammed into me but that would hardly have given the child immunity, so I just winced and cringed as I watched it violate her perfect flesh. My baby, of course, screamed at the peak of her voluminous lungs as the injection pierced her skin. I was sure she could be heard yelling miles away. She would not be comforted and stop crying. At least I knew this time why she was howling, I consoled myself as I rocked her. The child screamed all the way home, as I bundled her out of the surgery and into her blue pram and trundled her home. People stared at us in the street, as if I was trying to murder the baby after abducting her from her rightful mother. Belle, Trinny's model daughter, had of course not even whimpered after her injection.

After each immunisation, the child was, naturally, grumpy and sickly for days and would not be comforted by anything. She seemed able to make herself vomit at will, as if in protest at what I, her mother, had made her endure. And she had to have so many injections: for diphtheria, for tetanus, for whooping cough; and drops for polio, too. She had to have her first at only two months old, her second a month later, then her third, a month after that. It seemed appalling to me that there were so many, but I wanted her "safe" so I went along with them all like the obedient woman I had been brought up to be.

Now that my baby was born, I really longed for my own mother's presence in a way I never had before. I often saw young mums pushing prams with women who were obviously their own mothers, and this made me realise for the first time how much I wanted her by my side. The "good" version of my mother, not the "bad". I felt so alone and excluded in my own little rapidly shrinking world. But I knew my desire was ridiculous. My mum lived fifteen miles away and had her own life, looking after my dad and my brothers. I had to learn to cope all on my own, as usual.

When the baby was nine weeks old, I took her to visit the school I worked at. I didn't want to: I didn't even feel capable of leaving the house or taking her into the local Spar on my own. But Maggie Burton, the school headteacher, kept phoning and asking how the child was, saying they were all *dying* to see us both. Finally, just to stop her pestering, I said I would bring the baby in that Friday lunchtime.

I had to get up early on the Friday morning, to get myself and the baby ready with extra care. I was painfully aware of how both our appearances would be scrutinised and commented upon. I dressed the child very fastidiously in the pink-flowered dress and matching knickers that my mum had bought her when she was born. I clothed myself in my favourite pink, floral summer dress. It was, thankfully, loose, and skimmed over the baby fat I had not yet lost. I'd thought my figure would simply spring back to how it was before the baby, and in this, as in so much else, I was to be cruelly disappointed. I had changed shape, there was no hiding it: my breasts had fallen; my waist had thickened; my stomach was so spongy I doubted if it would ever be flat again. I did my best to hide my body with corrective (that is tight) underwear, but feared I was now such a podgy mess that I might never look attractive again. But, nevertheless, I continued with my damage limitation exercise, putting my contact lenses in for the first time since the child was born. They felt odd, gritty and irritating. I hoped they didn't make my eyes red and watery: I didn't want people to think motherhood had turned me into a crying, emotional wreck, which, of course, it *had.* I even wore my full make-up and jewellery. I felt like I was getting ready to go on stage to perform and, in a sense, I was. I surveyed myself in my bedroom mirror: it didn't look or even feel like me. Where had this stranger come from? I didn't look like I had before the baby. I didn't look "normal" somehow. Why was I leading this peculiar half-life where nothing was done or achieved and I just plodded on, feeling exhausted? I had no answers and neither did the odd woman in the mirror. I stared into her perplexed eyes but then the child started yelling again, so it was time to go.

I parked outside the school, a modern, small building for infants, all brick with large windows glinting, my heart beating hard with apprehension. I felt as anxious as if I was going for a job interview: what would I do if the baby was sick (likely) or cried (even more likely). I just didn't know what to do. Why didn't babies come with instruction manuals? The child was sure to embarrass me, and it would only serve to prove to everyone I used to know what a truly *useless* mother I was. At the same time, I felt so absolutely drained with the effort of getting ready (and all my medication was slowing me down, especially the antidepressants) that all I really wanted was for the child to sleep and then I could lie down and rest, too. The back seat of my black Fiesta looked impossibly inviting. But I psyched myself up into getting out of the car and, carrying the baby in her car-seat-cum-carrier, staggered into the school.

Tina, the smiley golden-haired secretary, was amazed to see me. 'I didn't know you were coming in!' she gasped. 'Why didn't you tell anyone you were coming?' 'I told Maggie,' I muttered. It seemed she had not told *anyone* else. She must have simply forgotten because she was so busy. But I did feel peculiar when everyone else was so surprised to see me. I felt like I had disappeared out of everyone's mind: that I had destroyed my career by having this child and now would never be accepted back into school life; that I had made my thorny bed and now must lie on it and not complain about the prickles.

I had hoped for a little friendly attention from my former work colleagues and, in this, as in everything else in my terrible life at that time, I was to be abundantly let down. They were all far too busy working.

Maggie had heard me talking to Tina by the reception desk and was there in an instant. She yelled, 'I'm so glad you've come to see us,' and hugged me for so long that my body went stiff. I didn't want this huge, theatrical fuss of me and the baby. I felt embarrassed. Maggie did want me back at work, I knew, because I was a good teacher with an excellent reputation in the school. She'd told me herself how often parents asked for their child to be put in my class. But I'd never thought that she liked me personally. Also, I was certainly not irreplaceable: who is? And we both knew it. Maggie ceremoniously presented the baby with some stuffed toys, and I thanked her.

But it was not Maggie I'd come to see. It was my former teaching colleagues I really wanted to talk with, especially the women who were mothers themselves. I longed for some reassurance from them that life did go on after having a child and that I too would, one day, return to "normal" and start living again. I did encounter a few of them as I wandered around the corridors but nobody else knew I was coming in and so they were all busy, teaching and preparing. One thing I did note was how shockingly confident everyone else was handling the baby. They passed her around in the staffroom at lunchtime as though she were a packet of digestives. They dandled her in their arms, on their laps and on their hips, as they sat or moved. I always held her as if she was made of easily broken Wedgwood and so I was always nervous around her. Equally appalling to me was the fact that they were all still talking about work, obsessed and engrossed in it: the national curriculum; SATS; assemblies; naughty children; clever children; OFSTED; other schools and job vacancies. I felt cast adrift. I had entirely lost touch with the world of work, its concerns and its specialised jargon. I felt as if my former colleagues were now talking a foreign language. I moved to my baby's rhythms alone now. My whole world had shrunk down to the few streets around my house, the newsagents, the dentist, the doctors, chemist and park. It was essentially just me and the child on stage with the odd walk-on guest appearance by Graham, the doctor, the nurse and my parents. How had my once enormous world shrunk so much and so quickly? What had happened to my life? I felt exiled onto a desert island when I used to be queen of the mainland.

 The few people I'd always liked best seemed genuinely glad to see me and I was pleased to see them, but something *had* happened, had altered irrevocably. They were part of something I no longer was, and I couldn't even conceive of getting back into it. The whole scene had shifted while I was looking the other way at the baby and now I'd missed my entrance cue. I no longer had a role in it and couldn't believe I ever would again. It was as if a plate of unbreakable glass had descended between me and my former work colleagues. How could I leave my child and go back to work? There was just so much organisation and effort involved with getting me and the baby ready and out of the house. It had been a massive and exhausting task simply to get us to the school today: and that was just to socialise for a couple of hours. How was I going to be able to teach all day and do my preparation and marking in the evening? There weren't enough minutes in twenty-four hours for all I had to do, to perform it as well as I did before. It seemed an insurmountable problem.

I stayed at the school from eleven thirty to one thirty, arriving just before my colleague's lunch hour, leaving just after. My whole visit had shimmered with such a strangely unreal quality to it. Sometimes I'd felt as if I was not physically there but was just watching the proceedings, like Scrooge, as an invisible ghost, revisiting my own past. It was all very odd. They had all gone back to teach when I said goodbye, feeling completely exhausted with a crotchety and restless baby. I let her snooze while strapped in her blue car-seat on the journey home. I was too tired to talk to her and keep her awake, even though I knew not talking to her would disrupt her sleep patterns yet again. This meant I would likely be up all night with her, measuring out my strides on the bedroom floor.

When I got home, I collapsed, bawling more loudly than the newly roused baby. Our tears mingled as I walked the living room floor, clutching her. I didn't even know why I was crying. Relief? Exhaustion? Regret? Fear? Really, it had gone well: the child had been unusually well-behaved and was much admired, but I was too detached to notice any of it. It was as if I'd watched the whole scene from above. I let the numbness wash over me and counted down the minutes until Graham got home.

Chapter 5

How would I manage?

On Thursday morning as I was changing the baby, I found a bright red smear of blood on her nappy. I thought my heart would stop beating. I rushed round to the doctor's again, hardly able to breathe. I waited over an hour to be seen in the crowded waiting room and each second dragged. It was absolute torture, trying desperately to keep the child quiet and amused, so that I didn't disturb the other elderly patients waiting. They all glared disapprovingly at me and the baby. Finally, a convulsive wreck, I got in to see the doctor. He reassured me that it was just bad nappy-rash and gave me some pink cream to rub on the baby's bottom. I felt distraught. How could the child have nappy-rash? I was changing her every four hours. I obviously should be doing it even more often. The bespectacled doctor didn't say so but that was probably what he was thinking. Maybe he would report me for neglect to the social services and they would take the baby off me? I slunk home, destroyed.

Lots of people have asked me how something so long desired, a baby, could so quickly turn into my worst nightmare. I can only repeat what abundant health professionals have told me – that postnatal depression is primarily caused by hormonal imbalances after childbirth. Thanks to ten years of fertility treatment and desperately trying to conceive, I was in the habit of noting my menstrual pattern very closely. I knew I was consistently on a normal twenty-eight to thirty-two day cycle, but after giving birth my periods became wildly irregular. I would bleed after twelve days, then after twenty-two, then after sixteen: there was no common sequence at all. In June, my doctor started me on a contraceptive pill. He thought it was just to regulate my menstrual cycle, but I was determined to make sure I did not get pregnant ever again. This would have been a miracle as I was certainly not having sex either, but I was taking no chances whatsoever. It was also at this time that we wrote to our fertility clinic giving them written legal permission to use our remaining frozen embryos in their research, so adamant was I that I did not want another child. So, it would be correct to say that my hormones were ricocheting around in turmoil, matching and affecting my thoughts, my moods and my emotions.

I've always kept a diary, and on the first of June, I noted: "I'm worried *sick* about going back to work." I do remember this well. I found teaching full-time extremely stressful. This was 1999. The government had introduced the national curriculum and was phasing in the literacy and numeracy hours. All planning, reports and record-keeping now had to be done on computers, not handwritten, and my information technology skills were then rather basic. These were the days when I always had at least thirty-two to thirty-four children in my class and no classroom assistants at all. The only help I could get was from parents I had to *beg* to come in to assist me. I was so very afraid I wouldn't be able to cope with my pressured, burdensome job and with such a demanding baby as well. It took me hours of a morning to get the child washed, fed, changed and dressed and ready myself, just to get out of the house for a quick walk. How would I manage? Graham told me I should go back to work for the last week of term in July and that way I'd get paid for the summer holidays. I knew we needed the money. We had the mortgage to pay; bills; the baby's expenses (a seven-day supply of disposable nappies alone cost more than we received in a week's child benefit). The next day I noted in my diary: "My mum told me I'd be better off at work, as I am a complete wreck." Thanks for that, Mum, typical of your usual helpful, supportive self, though I recorded that I laughed at this, acknowledging that she was right. It's obvious the anxiety about coping with full-time teaching as well as the baby seemed to come along immediately with the chaotic hormones.

So far, so normal, I'm sure. I seemed to be coping, though I felt like a fraud. My diary entry for the third of May states boldly: "Stopped taking the antidepressants." I think I know why I did this, although, of course, with hindsight, it was a foolish thing to do. I hate taking medication for anything, anyway. I'd always rather struggle on, despite pains and aches and not take anything for them. My mum had taught me this. Also, I must have felt I was better and more able to manage. I noted in my diary that in the evening of that day: "We drank champagne on the patio with Mum and Dad." This must have been to celebrate the baby's birth, as we were not in the habit of drinking champagne or anything much for that matter. I knew I couldn't drink alcohol on top of antidepressants, as it is dangerous. I must have felt I'd been through a terrible time in those first few hard weeks and now I deserved to relax, to try to get back to normal, as I was before I got pregnant with the baby. I must have told Doctor Singh as it's in his letter to Doctor Howson that I "stopped taking antidepressants and suffered a relapse."

The third of August was the first day I remember seriously wanting to kill myself. I'd been to visit my parents and I'd collected the baby's special white outfit, ready for her christening, that Sunday. I was driving home along the main double carriageway feeling tired as I always did. I knew I didn't want to go home. I was exhausted and there was so much to do in the house. Yet the baby stopped me from doing anything, so much so, going home felt like voluntarily slipping on a straitjacket. To choose to be in the house all alone with the baby felt like being tortured. She was dozing and would wake up grouchy, so I fully expected to be up all night with her, as usual, walking around her room like a half-dead shell of a person, fatigued beyond endurance. I remember staring at the brown brick walls along the side of the road as I sped past, when the thought popped into my mind: "Why not drive fast into the wall and end it all, right now?" It would simply be regarded as a sad accident and then no awkward questions would be asked. It felt so seductively easy. It would be the cessation of all my problems, of everything. Sweet endless rest and peace and no more torment. I recall gripping the wheel so tightly that my knuckles went white. I knew with just one sharp turn of the wheel I could do it: I really could. I felt so tempted. It was so attractive an impulse, almost irresistible. But I did resist it, somehow. This was *not* the way out, I told myself, repeatedly.

    I was drenched with sweat all over when I arrived home, my clothes soaked through. I did not dare to drive alone with Natalie for years after that.

The baby was constantly crying and poorly. She always vomited back one entire bottle every single day; she continually seemed to have a red runny nose from a cold; she was eternally yelling. She even had terrible cradle cap – these thickly encrusted yellow flakes on her head which just would *not* go, no matter what product I bought from the chemist to eradicate it. Daily, I grew ever more anxious and depressed about my difficult, sickly child. She was always so ill. How could I possibly leave her to go back to work? The date of my expected return loomed over me and got ever nearer, causing me to despair. I just did not know how I was going to cope. Mum had always said my entire married life that she would look after the baby when I returned to work, but I'd have to get the baby to her house. The child needed so many things with her every day: bottles; powdered milk; bottlebrush; steriliser; nappies; changing mat; wipes; nappy bags; bibs; clothes; change of clothes for when she was sick; pram; blankets; toys... the list seemed endless. How could I cram all of this into my black Fiesta and who would look after the child while I did it? To get to school by eight-thirty, I'd have to get up at five to get myself and the baby ready, load the car and get her to my parents' house. To wake up at five and have enough sleep, I'd have to be in bed by nine. When would I do all my marking and preparation? It was impossible! No wonder all these celebrities had a live-in nanny or two. That way, you could just leave the baby to the nanny (or an obliging granny, like some lucky mothers) and concentrate on getting yourself ready before rushing off to work. But the cost of a live-in nanny was astronomical. I'd probably have to pay her more than I was earning myself. And she'd expect to get her own car and time off and would she be any good? There was no guarantee. She'd probably be like that very expensive cleaner my friend Jane had once employed who'd turn up, watch her television, drink her Nescafé, eat all her ginger nuts and then demand her extortionate wages. It was like being mugged in her own home, she complained to me. Plus, I seemed to have no time or energy to sort out these problems. Just minute by minute, hour by hour, living exhausted me.

We all thought it was time the baby should be christened. I used to go to St. John's every Sunday and had done for the ten years I'd lived in the village. I was so anxious at this time that my skin kept breaking out into bloodied suppurating inflammations. I had delicate, sensitive skin and had been prone to eczema all my life.

At times of nervous anxiety it blazed up, but generally I kept it under control with the use of creams and oily baths. When I was trying to organise the christening my skin broke out more badly than ever before. The incessant itch drove me demented and the constant urge to scratch, and find some relief, was hard to ignore. I tried everything but nothing seemed to help. I went to the doctor one scorching hot day when even the high street shimmered in a heat haze like it was a beach in the south of France. I felt like I was physically part of that waiting room I'd been there so often, but at least I had a proper appointment and I had Graham with me to help entertain the baby this time. I got even more cream to put on top of my scarlet, weeping blisters.

'The doctor's always say the same thing,' I complained to Graham, when I came out. 'They always say, "Is anything bothering you?" Meanwhile, you sit there, your whole body one red, running sore, looking like The Elephant Man's uglier cousin and yet they say, "Is anything bothering you?"' Graham smiled at my sarcasm, but it was tempered by concern. He was very worried about me, he told me later. When I wasn't lethargic, I seemed permanently angry at everything. Having a child had altered my nature. Either that or the experience of it had brought the "real" me to the surface.

I planned the christening rather haphazardly and without enthusiasm. Before I was pregnant, I had discussed the occasion with Graham, just as we'd fantasised about every special event to do with our longed-for child. We had attended numerous christenings of other people's children and always noted the details: how the service went; what the babies were called (often the origin of great amusement); what the parents and godparent's wore; what hymns were sung; where the christening parties were held. In the same way soon-to-be-wed couples attended lots of weddings, so that they could plan their own and make it the best it could be. I had fondly imagined I'd visit all the designer shops in Liverpool, Manchester and Southport before choosing my carefully coordinated outfit, complete with matching hat, shoes, bag and gloves. I'd envisaged that I would scour the exclusive baby clothes shops for the perfect christening outfit for the child.

But the reality couldn't have been more different. I just didn't have the time or energy to be bothered. I bought my blue dress (with no matching anything) by pulling the first one I could reach off the rack at Marks & Spencer. I didn't even try it on as the baby was wailing loudly and growing so red in the face that passers-by were staring and nudging each other. I picked the christening gown out of a little catalogue that my dad gave me to look at. I paid him the money and he procured it from some obscure back street shop near where he used to work. It wasn't really what I had in mind but it was the easiest thing to do. I let the vicar choose the hymns: I simply didn't care. The baptism of my child, so eagerly anticipated, had turned into just something else I had to get through, another chore to add to the endless list.

Chapter 6

Dream crashed into nightmare

The actual day of the christening, Sunday the eighth of August, was yet another dream that crashed into a nightmare. I was feeling really tired yet made a superhuman effort to get myself and the baby ready on time before Graham drove us to St. John's. All my family and friends had already arrived apart from my older brother, John, who was as always late. (I didn't exactly care and only paid attention when he did finally turn up because my mum was so obviously furious, hissing and glaring at him). I didn't feel glad to see anyone. I just felt exhausted. Our baby started screaming the second she entered the church and kept up her wailing all through the entire ceremony, as if she were a demon-child possessed by the devil who couldn't bear such proximity to the divine. This was all my fault, as usual: I kept the house deathly quiet; no radio, no television, no music on at all, hoping the baby would fall asleep. She was, therefore, used to hardly any noise, so even the slightest sound frightened her and the blaring organ in the church must have terrified her so much that she couldn't help bawling. Yet one more thing to add to the long list of failures. I kept desperately trying to do the right thing, but just like in the nightmare that my life was turning into, it always kept turning out to be the wrong thing.

I'd been to over a hundred christenings, most at this very church but I had never known any child to behave as badly or yell as noisily as my baby. Even in my almost catatonic depressed state I felt so ashamed I just wanted to run out of St. John's, away from everyone and everything, especially my dreadful child. I was fantasising about behaving like the bride at the end of *The Graduate* where she leaves the church for another man, only in my version it was the baby's mother leaving the christening and running away on her own shouting, "Free at last!"

I hardly heard one word of the service and neither did anyone else because my baby's screaming, crying and whingeing drowned out everything else. There were three other children being christened at the same time and several of the guests had brought along video cameras to record the unique event, including my own brother Richard, but everyone had to switch their sound off because my child's endless shrieks were so ear-shattering. She ruined it for everyone. The other three babies were well-behaved and scarcely whimpered. Naturally, the very best of all was Belle, breath-taking and beautiful in armfuls of white silk and real lace, eclipsed only by her mother Trinny, dressed in a designer-chic royal blue suit with matching hat, shoes, bag and gloves. The whole service was obviously torture for everyone unfortunate enough to be present but especially agonising for me. I just wanted everything to stop so I could find some peace and quiet again, but the day just dragged on, infinitely. The child would not be quiet or comforted; nothing worked to muffle or stop the appalling din. I was sure I wasn't the only person in church who thought the vicar might crack and *drown* the baby in the font, finally putting an end to the awful, nerve-grating racket of her howling. I could barely glimmer a real smile for the photographs when, at last, the dreadful, interminable ceremony ended.

We had the party afterwards at our local pub, The Black Bull. I had wanted it to be at The Grand, the posh hotel opposite the church, but when we inquired we found it had already been booked by Trinny for Belle's ultra-glamorous christening party. Graham had expected the party to be at our house, but I had very firmly rammed down my size five shod foot against that ludicrous suggestion.

'I am NOT inviting anyone to the house,' I told him, unequivocally. 'I simply haven't the time or the energy to clean the house and prepare all the food.' As it was, I'd been so out of it in Greggs that I'd given them the wrong date for the christening, telling them the eighth of July (our wedding anniversary) rather than the eighth of August and there it was, iced in pink on top of the cake. I'd hoped nobody would notice but, of course, everybody delighted in pointing it out to me, making me feel even more inadequate.

At the party I hardly spoke to anyone, nor could I eat anything. I just sat and stared venomously at everyone in resentment. The baby, worn out by her relentless, raging tantrum in church, was sleeping tranquilly in her blue pram which meant she'd be up all night again, keeping me awake, too. I glared at her sleeping so serenely and felt no tenderness. If any passing raggle-taggle strangers had wanted to take the baby there and then, I would have thankfully given her away without a pang of guilt. Adoption was the only sensible solution, but how could I get Graham to agree to it? He seemed to think I'd been joking when I mentioned it to him, but I had never been more deadly serious in my entire life.

The christening had been my one opportunity to show everyone what I had after everything I'd suffered. It was supposed to have been my vindicating moment, my time on the world stage to proclaim, "Yes, I *know* I've destroyed my life, my health and my career but look what I have instead: a wonderful baby. Just see how happy I am." But the child had taken my moment of triumph from me and spoilt it, just like I felt she'd ruined my entire life. I glowered at the baby and sulked. I just wanted to go home to rest and close the door on the world, especially my own daughter.

On the Saturday after the dreadful christening, we had arranged to go to Smile Please! the local photographer's studio, for an official christening portrait. This was yet another of my cherished fantasies that was about to turn into a bad dream. In other people's homes I had frequently admired the family photographs exhibited, often shining glossily, showing the wife, husband and child all elatedly smiling yet relaxed, the very epitome of "Happy Family". This was exactly what I wanted for myself: a trophy for our walls and the walls of our loved ones.

Naturally it did not work out that way at all. We dressed in our christening outfits, me in my ill-fitting, too-light-blue dress and old jacket; Graham in his blue blazer and white-spotted navy tie; the baby in her cheap white polyester christening gown, matching bootees and bonnet. We sat awkwardly on the photographer's couch and tried, in vain, to look like a "proper" family. I sat the baby on my knee and tried to calm her down to stop her from yelling but she wriggled so much, she could hardly even keep her bootees on her squirming feet or her bonnet on her jerking head. I felt deeply uneasy, like I was trying to settle and arrange a giant *squid* on my lap. I really should have taken her off into a murky corner beforehand and grappled with her until she capitulated. Even Graham felt uncomfortable and edgy, knowing that the baby might start screaming or be sick at any moment, aware of how depressed and anxious I was feeling. It's an often repeated saying that the camera never lies, and it was true, in this case: there it was, in plain sight for anyone to see, I thought. The resultant photograph, which cost us a fortune, and was put up in our house and the grandparents' houses and all the houses of the godparents, aunties, uncles, cousins and friends. It was absolutely appalling. And we could never get away from it, as it was everywhere we went and every single time I caught the momentary sight of it, I felt sick and wanted to fling it on the floor and grind it under my stiletto heel, crushing it into dust. It perfectly captured the disordered state of my mind at that dreadful time. My strange face told the whole sorry story: I didn't want to be there: I didn't even want to be alive on this earth. I have a fake, tense, half-formed expression on my pale face that is meant to be a smile and dismally fails. My eyes look *dead.* I had withdrawn from the present to a much darker place. I look like a persecuted soul crying out for assistance but all I could do was sit there and pretend to be part of a happy family. The baby looks exactly like the cheeky, wriggling, demanding imp that she was, her left bootee hanging off, white dress all squiggly around her, creased, mouth poised, ready to yell. Graham looks prematurely old, grey and lined; even he cannot smile properly. He looks worried, apprehensive and false. Afterwards, I could never bear to look directly at this photograph and loathed its ubiquity, wanting every copy destroyed. But there they all remained, mocking me, a constant reminder that there was a time in my life when I should have been at my most happy, but I had been robbed of this state and just wanted to *die.* One more cherished ambition had crashed into yet another bad dream.

The child was now five months old and therefore ready to move onto solid food and mashed-up fruit. I tried incessantly, purchasing a blender to whizz ingredients together, buying every make of baby food, every concoction possible, organic and non-organic, household name and obscure brand but the outcome was always the same: the baby would not open her mouth for the food and if, by chance, I tricked her and managed to sneak a spoonful in between her ready-to-clamp gums, she invariably *spat* it out, a look of passionate disgust on her fiendish features. I told the health visitor, but she didn't seem to think it was a problem.

'She looks well enough,' the woman pronounced. But I thought the baby looked ill, pale and scrawny, with flame-coloured hair to match her temper tantrums. I was in despair. The child would not eat, she would not sleep, she vomited back all her milk: she was going to *die,* and it was completely my fault for being such a hopeless mother and now I had to go back to work. It was a perfect storm of *horror.*

I had somehow gone back to work in July for the last week of term and it had been terrible. I felt like I was sleep-walking through it, shell-shocked and shaken. And that had been after I'd begged my mum to stay in our house, to look after the baby and I didn't have my own class to take. Now it was time for me to go back to work properly, to start in September and take a whole new reception form and manage all on my own. I was incredibly anxious, agitated and not sleeping or eating much at all. I walked around the house, not able to relax, pressing my hands together to stop them shaking. I was due back on the 6th of September, the class-lists had been distributed; the parents and children had been told I was to be their class teacher. But how, in god's name was I supposed to do it? How was I going to cope with the pressure of a stressful and demanding job on top of the strain from a worrying and exactingly difficult baby? Every time I had a moment to open my planning sheets, all the black words seemed to *jiggle* about on the white page and get mixed up with each other. This is what it must be like to be dyslexic, I thought. I could hardly read a line, never mind write one. I felt simultaneously too tired and anxious, and I had to be ready to teach on the 7th of September. I had always prided myself on my preparation for my new class. I had always shown up for that first day of school with all my planning and preparation done, all the children on my class-list sorted into groups, a seating plan ready, name badges made, their names written on the front of all their books and planning records. But now there just wasn't time with all I had to do for the baby. My mind, which used to be sponge-like when absorbing anything had turned into a repelling magnet, so that I could not seem to retain anything. It was like an off switch had been flicked in my head and my memory just didn't work anymore.

I told Graham and he thought I should go to see the doctor again. He took me on the 12th of August, leading me decisively by the hand, on a day so dazzlingly radiant it made me squint. This time I was lucky. I saw Doctor Howson, the only woman doctor at the group practice and I immediately felt the welcome warmth, sympathy and kindness radiating from her. At last, an empathic woman I could talk to! After listening to me talking hesitantly for fifteen minutes, she put me on a higher dose of the antidepressants the other doctor had started me on, after the baby was born. In my diary I've written that I didn't sleep at all on the night of Saturday the 14th of August. By Sunday I was in such a state of anxious agitation that Graham was seriously worried about me. He made me promise to see Doctor Howson again, the next day, which I did, and she told me I would have an appointment to see a psychiatrist and I must *not* be left alone with the baby. My diary entries are peppered with, "Phone Tina: are the books in yet?" These were the large blank books that the children did most of their work in. I always divided those in my new class into red, green, blue and yellow ability groups, based on what the nursery staff said about them, in the summer break and wrote their names on the covers of all their books. There was quite a technique to it, as the headteacher liked it done in a very particular way and it took hours to do all the different books for the whole class of thirty-two, which was why I was keen to do it before starting back at school, when there would be a hundred other things to do and quickly. I remember I became quite obsessed with getting these books and was constantly frustrated as Tina said there were none in stock though on order. I also became overly concerned with the baby's feeds, making notes and lists of them and with housework as detailed in my admission notes from the psychiatric hospital. The cleaning was a ritual, 'by which I was to keep the baby alive,' I told Doctor Singh, who noted it under "delusions and obsessions."

My anxiety about the baby had taken over my life by this point and completely unbalanced me: the fear of going back to work finished me off. I was barely coping with looking after the child. I knew I couldn't manage such a stressful and demanding job as well. I needed a rest, not more strain on top of the extreme stress I was already experiencing. I've always been described as very conscientious. Every school report I've ever had mentions this about me. I hated doing anything wrong or letting anyone down, and now I knew I was about to in the worst possible and most enormous way.

On the 26th of August I had an appointment with Doctor Howson. She was very concerned at my state and told me I was *not* to go back to work. She gave me a sick note for four weeks and increased the antidepressants again from 30mgs to 40mgs. I must have felt some relief that I would miss the terribly pressurised beginning of the school year, but I knew it was just that one of my many problems had merely been deferred. I was constantly hearing music playing in my head now, but this was much more pleasant and less painful than the demanding voices. It was all sixties and seventies hits from my teenage years, a golden era when music was incredibly important to me, mainly Tamla Motown singles with "Baby" in the title. *Baby Love* was one such typically apposite song that played on continually in my head. I really thought, and I must have told this to Doctor Singh as it's in his initial assessment notes and his letter to Doctor Howson, that my brain was playing me familiar songs to try to relax and soothe me. I needed to be calmed down as I was writing lists obsessively on the baby's sleeping and eating habits and noting how often I changed her nappy. I was also checking on the child constantly as she slept, feeling sure and frightened that she was going to *die* and, paradoxically terrified that I was going to be the one who killed her. I told my psychiatrists and nurses and anyone else who would listen, repeatedly, that I was a bad mother. Nobody bothered to contradict me. How could they? I so obviously was.

On the 7th of September I had my worst panic attack yet, as I waited over an hour to see Doctor Howson. I really thought I was dying. I was shaking all over, having heart palpitations and I could not breathe. She was very disturbed when she saw me and told me I only had to wait the minimum length of time to see her in the future. On the 9th of September my diary states that I saw Doctor Herald and Doctor Rahman. I recognise the names as those of two psychiatrists I saw regularly after I was discharged from psychiatric hospital. Doctor Rahman was Doctor Singh's deputy at the hospital, and came to my house with him on the 21st of September. Bizarrely, I can't remember one single thing about this interview, not even where it was held, surely an example of extreme stress affecting my mental processes adversely. They must have thought I was coping all right as they didn't do anything about me at this time. I must have still been able to hold my life together before it came so disastrously crashing down. All this time I was cleaning obsessively in an insane attempt to keep the baby alive, and I still could not seem to eat anything. Any food I put in my mouth felt like it was expanding and becoming so dry that I could hardly swallow it. In the two weeks before I was admitted to hospital, I lost over half a stone, as detailed in my medical notes.

I was getting worse. I noted in my diary that every day Graham took the baby to his mother's house where a childminder called Lorraine looked after her, paid by Graham's mum. One day Lorraine was sick, so he left the child at his sister Janet's house, and she took the day off work to care for the baby, as it was an emergency. This was the time when Doctor Singh wrote in his notes that I had nothing to do with the child at all: I was not bonded with her, felt numb towards her and blamed her for the awfulness of my dreadful half-life, jealous that Graham seemed to love and enjoy our daughter and I did not. I was crying, weepy, tired and morbid, the doctor reported.

The antidepressants did not seem to be working. They just made me feel tired. I had to fight the exhaustion all the time. I had so much to do and so few minutes in the day and felt like I was trudging through black treacle. I thought that my own body and my own baby were persecuting me, and felt tortured by the child as if the anchors of my sanity, time and place, were gradually becoming untied. There seemed to be no such thing as day or night, normal patterns of eating or drinking, waking or sleeping. Everything was tangled together and distorted. I was constantly tired, hungry, sore, uncomfortable, distressed and, most of all, afraid: there was no routine and my mind craved one. I was terribly frightened of the black unknown: what would be my future? What had happened to my life? How would I survive?

The insistent voices in my head seemed to make so much sense. Pain was everywhere, crowding in on me. I couldn't even watch the news any more or flick through *The Guardian* because the voices lurked there, too, telling me that all these terrible things in the news were about to happen to me and my baby: mothers and children were being hurt, maimed, raped and violated: me and my child were next. It was as if I'd shed my outer layer of skin, like a boa-constrictor, and now all my protection was gone. I was in such a heightened state of sensitivity that all the barriers between my own pain and other peoples had broken down and been dissolved so that I felt everything: all this hurt was pushing against me, incessantly. I had to *kill* the baby first, release her from all her agony. Why else did she cry all the time if she wasn't in constant, unremitting torment, like her mother? Next, I had to *kill myself* and then we would both be out of it, freed and not have to feel all this torturous suffering anymore. This was what I HAD to do. I had no choice. It was for the best. It would be sad, obviously, but what else could I do? It was the only way out.

I stood by the baby's cot for hours listening to her breathe, looking at her downy arms circled around the bright red hair on her head, watching her innocently dreaming, her impish face blushing a pink glow, wondering how best to kill her. Suffocation would be the easiest way, I decided. It would not take much pressure. I would just put the pillow over her little pouting mouth: it would be like a huge snowflake whirling down from heaven; she probably wouldn't even cry; it would be just like going to sleep. 'Go to sleep my baby, close your little eyes.' The lullaby lilted in my mind as I stood by the cot, which made a pleasant change from *Baby Love* and all the other sixties and seventies pop songs my mind was constantly playing me nowadays. If she whimpered a little, as I pressed the pillow down over her face, I would whisper to her: 'Mummy's here. It's all right. This is our way out: trust me!' I could see the brightness of the end blaze clearly now. It was the only reasonable option, I told myself once again. I could picture the heap of paracetamol and antidepressants I'd been hoarding on my bedside table with a glass of water, waiting invitingly. 'Soon I'll join you,' I wanted to croon. 'You won't be alone, I promise you, my little darling. We'll be together now forever, and nobody will hurt us ever again. My sweetheart, this is how much Mummy loves you. She'll do *anything* for you, really anything…'

Graham walked into the bedroom. 'Everything all right?'

'Yes. You're back from the chippy quickly.'

'Yes. Nobody in as normal for a Monday. Why are you staring at the baby?'

'It's okay,' I told him, my voice tired. 'I just have to kill the baby and then myself. The voices keep telling me to…' I looked at him but did not get the reassurance I sought.

'It's not okay.' He spoke very clearly, as if to a child. 'What are these voices saying?'

'The voices are saying I have to kill the baby. They keep saying, "The baby must die," over and over again and then, "You must die."'

'Lorna, you're not well.' Graham's voice was strange, low but urgent, almost pleading. 'I'm going to get you some help. It's okay. Everything is going to be fine.' He guided me out of the room.

I sat on the sofa in the living room, hearing his voice on the telephone in the hall. He was talking intently but I couldn't hear what he was saying. Graham thought I wasn't well.

I knew things were not the way they should be but what could I do about it? I was so exhausted; I could hardly think or feel.

Chapter 7

Danger to yourself and others

Graham got me an emergency appointment with Doctor Howson for the next day. 'You *must* tell her about the voices,' he urged me, as he left. He took the child to work with him, dropping her off at his parents' house where Lorraine, the childminder, looked after her. He was seriously worried about me, and didn't know what was going on in my mind anymore. Before the baby was born we talked all the time. We had made all sorts of special plans and shared everything together. Only now did he realise how very little I'd been saying to him. He knew I felt rather depressed and uneasy, not sleeping well and wondering how to cope but surely most new mothers felt that way? He felt like that himself! But I seemed to be getting worse, not better, even though I was taking a course of antidepressants. The doctor who'd visited when the baby was first born told him he thought it should be best practice for *all* new mothers to be prescribed antidepressants. But Graham had been incredibly disturbed when I told him I was hearing voices in my head, telling me to *kill*. Surely only severely crazy people like schizophrenics heard such voices. He hoped Doctor Howson could help me.

The next day I was waiting in the doctor's surgery. I remember just sitting there, staring down at the beige floor, not able to think or even care.

My name was called, and I went in.

'How are you feeling now, Lorna?' Doctor Howson asked as I sat down.

'Perhaps I should increase the dosage of your antidepressants?' Before he left the house with the baby that morning, Graham had reminded me to tell the doctor about the voices.

I sighed, as talking took so much effort. 'I keep hearing voices telling me to kill the baby and myself...' I managed.

Doctor Howson's gentle face instantly changed expression from sympathy to consternation, her blue eyes glistening. 'Lorna, *how* do you hear these voices?'

'They're in my head telling me what to do... they go on and on,' I sighed. 'I just want them to stop.'

'What do they say?'

'The baby *MUST DIE! You MUST DIE!*'

'Lorna,' Doctor Howson's face and tone were very serious now. 'I really think you may need to go into hospital to get the help you need. I'm going to ask two doctors and a social worker to come and visit you at home.'

'I don't mind.' I started to shrug but gave up, as it required too much exertion. 'It doesn't matter. Nothing matters.' I breathed out deeply. I really didn't care if I lived or died.

Doctor Howson immediately reached for her phone.

Later at home when some time had passed, I heard my front door-bell chime. I opened the silver-framed glass door to find three strange people lurking outside. They all came rushing at me with their long coats flapping like the wings of huge, black crows. They looked as if they were ready to pick over their carrion and I was their prey. Then my panic subsided, and I saw they were just two men and one woman. The man with the charismatic, smiling unlined face seemed to be in charge. I liked him right away which was unusual for me as I'm usually cautious about new people.

'I am Doctor Singh,' he told me softly, proffering his hand. I shook it automatically. He seemed engagingly cheerful and had kind, twinkling brown eyes. 'This is my colleague, Doctor Rahman.' He, too, stepped forward to shake hands. He had a fascinatingly tragic face and sad, almost black eyes. 'And this is Elaine Moore, an approved social worker.' The woman, too, stepped forward to grin and shake hands. 'May we come in?' asked the first doctor.

I ushered them into the hall and then into the living room. We all sat down. I perched on my brown sofa. Doctor Singh had the gentlest manner possible. I simply couldn't imagine him upsetting anybody, ever. He asked me questions, as if I was a new friend he was eager to get to know better, finding everything I said, however mundane, fascinating. He glowed with intuition and sensitivity, and I trusted him at once.

Graham walked in, home from work, carrying the baby. He looked shocked to find his own living room full of strangers. Everyone was introduced to him, and they all shook hands.

'Why do we need *two* doctors?' he asked the social worker, quietly.

'It takes two doctors to section someone under the Mental Health Act,' she replied, in a matter-of-fact manner.

Graham had to turn his face away, shocked and sickened. He knew I needed medical help and that things could not continue as they had; but to *section* me? It was like something out of a Victorian Gothic horror novel, locking the mad woman away in the mental asylum. He half-expected to see a straitjacket with leather straps and chains poking out of the doctor's briefcase. He consoled himself with the thought that they were all experienced, qualified health professionals: they must have known what they were doing.

The social worker approached him. 'Shall I take the baby now?' she asked, arms outstretched.

Graham automatically tightened his grip on the child. 'Take the baby where?' he gasped.

'I'll take the baby with me, into care. She'll be well looked after. All our care homes and foster parents are under constant scrutiny…'

'No, no,' spluttered Graham, shaking his head thinking that this was even worse than he'd imagined. 'We'll manage to look after the baby… between us, as we have been doing. I've got Lorna's parents and mine and my sister… We'll cope.' He hugged the child close and took her to my side, but I seemed sadly oblivious.

I felt like I wasn't really *there,* strangely quite conscious of what was happening all around me but oddly unaware that any of it applied to me.

Graham realised that the doctors were in the middle of assessing me so he waited outside, walking up and down the hall with the baby pressed to his heart, sick with worry.

Doctor Singh carried on asking me questions. I answered as truthfully as I could: how I felt about the child and my life; what the voices had been telling me to do; how I planned to kill the baby and myself. I replied to his neutrally phrased questions prosaically, like an automaton, yet they were heavy with meaning. Graham told me later he felt like he was the only real, emotional human being in the house. Doctor Singh was asking these weighted questions so dispassionately and noting down the outrageous answers without any response at all, like he was asking about the weather, and I was saying it might rain later but would soon clear up. And I seemed completely drained of feeling, as if I'd given up on my life and didn't care. Where was the woman he loved? Graham asked himself.

I wasn't even aware that he was there when he came back into the living room, though he said he was staring at me, willing me to look back at him. Everything was too painful, so I had withdrawn deep inside like I was closing myself down, getting ready to die. The flame of life that used to burn so brightly within me had dwindled until it was barely flickering, like a pilot-light in a central heating boiler, about to go out. I felt so close to death; just millimetres away; I merely had to stretch out my hand and I would cross that line. I wanted to die and be extinguished for good. My inner flame of spirit had not been nourished: it had been stifled, then starved and now I felt as if a faint puff of breath could blow me over into that other world. It was nobody's fault. I was more than ready to die. My life was over. It wasn't important and I didn't care. Nothing mattered. *I was completely lost.*

Graham waited outside while I was questioned further. He was relieved to see my parents arrive. He had phoned them as soon as it was mentioned that I would be sectioned and admitted to psychiatric hospital. He rushed to greet my mum and dad, so happy to see that other human beings had now landed on Planet Disturbed Yet Emotionless.

'I think Lorna has to go into hospital, as I told you on the phone,' Graham paused, saddened to see their faces crease with worry. 'Can you look after the baby while I drive her there?'

'Of course, we'll look after the child,' my mum told him. She later told me that I didn't seem at all bothered and it was Graham she felt sorry for, as he looked so shell-shocked and lost.

They came into the living room and I looked up, feeling vaguely surprised to see my mum and dad, wondering why they were there. I made that trying-to-smile-but-can't grimace that I wear in the infamous, hated christening portrait. My parents responded with polite, social, invited-to-dinner smiles rather than broadcast the full horror of what they felt.

Doctor Singh took numerous notes and filled in myriad rainbow-coloured forms that Doctor Rahman then countersigned. He now stopped writing and looked at me directly, fixing me in his brown-eyed beam. I sensed that what he was about to say must be important and so I tried to concentrate. 'Lorna May Davies,' he told me, 'I consider you to be a danger to yourself and to other people, as does my colleague Doctor Rahman and therefore, unless you agree to be admitted to psychiatric hospital voluntarily, I will section you under the Mental Health Act of 1983 and you will have no choice.'

I bowed my head in acknowledgement of my sentence from my strange judge.

'What's the difference between being sectioned and *not* being sectioned?' asked Graham. He sounded upset but I had no idea why.

Doctor Singh shrugged. 'Nothing really: an informal admission just means fewer forms for us to fill in.'

But something, the words, the tone or the atmosphere had penetrated the black, blanket-like fog all around me and I knew this was deadly serious. 'I will enter hospital voluntarily,' I said. I sensed vaguely that things were not right and that I needed help. I went upstairs to pack a suitcase, rather distractedly, not knowing what to take or how much, unaware of how long I would be in hospital. Surely, I wouldn't be in for a lengthy time? I just bundled a few clothes, some underwear, my toothbrush and sponge bag into my old tan-coloured case. I had heard, 'Twenty-eight days,' spoken aloud but didn't realise it applied to me: that this was the *least* amount of time I would definitely be in the psychiatric hospital for assessment and treatment. Would it have made any difference to me, if I'd known for how long I was to be incarcerated? Not really, I realised, afterwards: I had finished with my life and was just waiting to die.

We all set off in a convoy to go to the hospital. I can't remember even kissing the baby or saying goodbye to her. I think I was completely indifferent to leaving her, like she had nothing to do with me and the same was true of how I left my parents. The two doctors went first with the social worker, in a shiny, black Jaguar. Was that where they kept the straitjackets and restraints? Graham thought, grimly. He tried not to think about what they might do to me. He followed in our car with me strapped in the passenger seat. He tried to guess what I was thinking but he could read nothing in my closed face. I had retreated far from him. Perhaps this strange hospital could bring me back?

I remember being surprised that it was night-time and very murky. Buildings seemed to loom at us out of the intense blackness. When did all this darkness fall? I had no idea. I didn't know where the hospital was; and I didn't care. Graham drove on for miles it seemed. I felt as if I was living on another level of existence where nothing that happened on this earthly plane affected me at all; only it wasn't a higher level of existence that saintly people lived on; it was a lower plane, below animal life, below plant life, below rock life, where nothing seemed to go on under my weighty, protective crust: I had become fossilised while I still lived.

I had met, at different times in my life, two people who had both gone on to take their own lives and had noticed this same strange thing about each of them. I had looked into their troubled eyes and they had both *closed* me out, they turned away; they didn't want to know. They were on their own where they thought nobody could help or reach them: suffering souls in isolation and close to welcoming death; sad, tortured people I had not known well. One was the older sister of a university friend; the other was a male friend of a work colleague.

I had met both only once, by chance, when I called on my friends, but I'd never forgotten that chillingly empty look in both pairs of eyes and that air of intense seclusion that hung around them like white mist. They had withdrawn completely and were waiting for death to take over. If I'd known them better and realised what it was, maybe I could have done something about it and helped them? But perhaps not: maybe they were beyond help. And perhaps I was past saving, too.

I could not bear to look in the mirror in case I had that very same look. I had lost my own self. I couldn't even think about what was going to happen to me.

Chapter 8

Dangerous remedies

We all arrived together in the car park at the hospital. It emerged out of the blackness – huge, dim and forbidding – only the ground floor was lit up, like a shop window. The doctors escorted us in. We all went up in a slow, indolent lift that chimed regretfully, a muted, "ding-dong" as it reached the first floor. I smelt the reek of disinfectant. We were conducted to "Mansfield," the female admissions ward. We were taken to the office where more people were waiting for us, and I was formally admitted to the psychiatric hospital. It was the 21st of September 1999, I was told. Two nurses asked me innumerable questions and filled in numerous forms. A male doctor checked me over physically. I felt as if all this was happening to someone else, not me. Then I was ushered, meekly, to my room and Graham left.

I was relieved to find that I had my own private room, number 26, the very first around the corner from the main corridor, where the office was situated. It even had its own bathroom, containing a shower cubicle and toilet, cunningly devised to fit in a triangular space, taking up one corner of my room. I was so glad I had not been put on a huge, public ward with the crazy lunatics! I did actually say this to my special named nurse. She wrote it in her intervention record: "Lorna was relieved to find the hospital was not an asylum full of axe-murderers." She didn't tell me what I found out later: they kept all the mad axe-murderers in the more secure unit next door! My first impression of my room was that it was surprisingly satisfactory like a basic, clean, newly-built hotel. Only gradually did I notice the small but telling details that proved it was, indeed, a psychiatric hospital. The glass in the window looked unbreakably thick, so I couldn't smash it or throw myself out to escape back home. I soon found out that the water in the shower, the taps of the basin and the few baths found down the corridor ran very slowly and noisily so it would be impossible to drown oneself. Even in the dining room, I discovered later, all the cutlery and beakers were plastic, so I couldn't slit my wrists or stab myself with it; or use it on anyone else. The mattress on my bed was covered on top with rubber that rustled when I lay on it to protect it if I wet myself (which the alcoholics did, regularly, I later found out.) At the four corners of my bed, I found loops of thick rubber, presumably restraints, to be used to hold me if I became violent. But these odd features I only noticed by degrees, as the black fog that swirled around my troubled mind slowly dispersed. My first reaction, as far as I could be bothered about anything, was that it was much better than I had feared, so I was relieved. I unpacked my few clothes and quickly buried them away in the chest-of-drawers and matching wardrobe. Then I lay on my crinkling bed and stared at the white ceiling. I had been told to attend supper at ten even if I wasn't hungry, because it was after this meal that the medication would be given out. 'If you try to miss this, we will come and fetch you,' I had been told by the nurses. I longed to curl up and doze throughout the whole winter, like a hibernating tortoise in a Blue-Peter-prepared cardboard box. I just wanted to go to sleep *forever*.

But I forced myself to stay awake. I had noticed that my room was the very first and nearest to the office, but I didn't detect the strange eyes checking on me every fifteen minutes through the spyglass in the door or know that this would continue all through the day and night. I had no idea at all that I was on fifteen-minute suicide watch. I only found out afterwards, when I was moved further away and no longer a high-risk "category three". I just lay on my bed gazing at the ceiling, wondering what was going to happen to me, wanting to be somewhere else.

I did keep checking my watch, to be on time for supper at ten. I didn't feel at all hungry, I just didn't want the humiliation of having the nurses come to fetch me. This had been told to me not as a threat but as a simple statement of fact and that was chilling. It was then that I half-realised that I now had no "rights" at all. I had been admitted to a psychiatric hospital and now all my civil liberties had been suspended, like I was a criminal or an "imbecile". It didn't help me now that my sense of self seemed to have disintegrated, nor that I found I was now in a sort of patriarchal state in which all the women patients had no rights, all the psychiatric nurses were female and did all the work and the only men around (apart from rare male visitors) were the God-like psychiatric consultants who had absolute power over everybody. Their edicts were law: one *word* from them and the women could be taken away for legal "torture" via electric shocks, a lobotomy, or taken to other "more secure" units, about which dark stories were whispered. Such rumours included tales of women hauled away, shrieking in straitjackets, at blackest night, chained up in padded cells, restrained and drugged for twenty-four hours a day, operated upon. Some even vanished. I saw no evidence of any of these things, but it is indicative of the anxiety we all had. Fear was the prevailing emotion I and all the other patients felt. In my anxiously heightened state, the hospital seemed even more sinister and frightening for being outwardly so normal, even luxurious. Only the inmates thought they knew what was really going on but who would believe any of us? We were all legally and officially *mad*. I felt like an enchanted medieval princess, lavishly entertained in the castle's great hall with feasting and entertainment, yet all along I was aware of the deep, dangerous dungeons in the castle's keep, where people were tortured and left to decompose, in rags and chains, stinking of their own vomit, urine and excrement as dragons lurked, hidden in their black lairs, waiting to be fed. It was more frightening in that I wasn't consciously able to vocalise my fears: I was tired and drugged. I had no idea what was going to happen to me or my life, and I felt too exhausted to care.

Nevertheless, at one minute to ten I dragged myself back to the office on the main corridor and found the dining room opposite all lit up. It contained a moving mass of sixty-or-so women, sitting on chairs or milling around. Some wore dressing-gowns over nightdresses, slippers on their feet, as if ready for bed. There were thick, white teacups and saucers stacked high on a big, wooden trolley with glinting chrome handles. The women helped themselves to tea or coffee out of enormous metal teapots. I realised, suddenly, that I was thirsty and just fancied a cup of tea, so I took my place in the queue, watched what to do and helped myself to the surprisingly heavy teapot to fill my cup. There were also cereal bowls full of various small packs of biscuits: bourbons; custard creams; garibaldi and digestives. Each packet contained only two or three. I took one of rich tea to fit in with the others but noticed some of the women took two or even three packets. Then they all went to sit around the tables, eating and drinking their supper.

I didn't know where to sit but a young girl with long, dark brown hair looked at me and smiled invitingly. Feeling relieved, I tried to grin back and sat on the empty seat next to her.

'Sometimes they make us toast,' she told me. 'If Gina was on, she'd make us toast but she's not working tonight. I'm Jodie, by the way.'

'I'm Lorna.' I managed to stretch my mouth into a turned-up shape again, but my face had got out of the practice of smiling and felt really strange. I was glad to see that Jodie seemed so "normal" – not that I knew what that was any more. I was content just to munch my biscuits and sip my lukewarm, stewed tea and look at all the vast variety of women there. Some looked like teenagers and others looked old and grey-haired, walking in a doddery fashion, and there was every age in between. Some were clothed ready for bed, which had surprised me at first, whereas others looked like they'd dressed with their eyes closed, arrayed in a random hotchpotch of garments. Two or three looked smartly chic as if they were ready for a shoot for the glossy pages of a fashion magazine.

I stared around, *bewildered,* at all these women, blinking under the harsh lights, wondering vaguely why they were all in there but too immersed in my own problems really to care. They all gobbled their biscuits and gulped their tea and coffee, talking and watching two of the nurses push an enormous wooden cabinet on wheels into the dining room and ceremoniously unlock it. I thought it was a mahogany writing bureau, but it turned out to be a medicine cabinet. It had a metal tray beneath it containing coloured files: green, red, blue and yellow. The duty nurse would pick up whichever coloured dossier had been left on top and work her way through them. She would find the first name in the folder and call it out and the patient would approach the trolley and take the little, white, plastic cup of pills offered. One nurse would give out the drugs and the other would check that the medication was correct and in the right dosage, and would give the patient a plastic tumbler of water out of the water dispenser, which was also on top of the cabinet. Both nurses watched carefully to check that the patient swallowed all the drugs there and then, in front of them. I soon learned they didn't just give out medication to control our various conditions. All the patients were asked by the nurses if they also needed any sleeping pills, painkillers, laxatives or even contraceptive pills: all were doled out, formally and cheerfully. It took a long time. Some few rebellious inmates questioned every single item of their medication, arguing, 'I don't have that!' or 'This is too high a dose!' But most, like me, just swallowed everything they were given, not knowing, asking or even caring what it was. The hardest thing, I found, was swallowing all my pills down in front of these sharply watchful strangers but I had to get used to it, like everyone else. Only when we had been seen to swallow *all* our medication where we allowed to go to bed, although a small group of patients seemed prepared to stay up late.

The same drug dispensing ritual was continued after breakfast, lunch and tea. I eventually realised that each coloured ring binder contained the names of all the patients under one particular consultant psychiatrist. I found out that my name was third in the red folder with the rest of Doctor Singh's patients so that was the one I waited for during the interminably long process of the drug dispensation.

I didn't know, at first, whether my cloudy mental state was because of my condition or because of the huge amount of medication I was given to "cure" it. Every Friday morning, I attended a case conference with Doctor Singh and his team, including some of the nurses on the ward, where my state was discussed and my medication often changed, altered, reduced or increased as I improved or deteriorated. At the beginning, according to my visitors (Graham; my parents; my brothers Richard and John and my vicar, Colin) I used to walk around like one of the living dead, with my arms outstretched in front, dragging my heavy legs after me. I also used to perspire a great deal, which I hardly ever did much before. When Graham questioned the nurses about this, he was told it was due to my excessive anxiety. (This was something he had noticed as soon as the baby was born. I changed from someone who hardly even glowed to someone who was constantly dripping with sweat. This sounds like a hormonal problem to me, closely associated with the night sweats and hot flushes of the menopause.) Then my sedatives were reduced, and I went through an agitated stage where my whole body, but especially my hands, would shake uncontrollably and inconveniently, like an old age pensioner with Parkinson's disease. Then I had a phase of pacing up and down. This was slowly brought under control, and I began to feel and act much more "normally" though I had every reason to lose faith in the whole concept of normality: who was to say what was normal and what was not? And why was it always *men* who decided how women should behave? I had once seen a film called *The Stepford Wives* about all these married American women living in a small town called Stepford. They all took their medication at a certain time of day, making them all happy, passive housewives, content just to look after their men and children and never to argue or divorce their husbands, no matter what they did. I felt like I was living in that film. Lunatic asylums and drugs were being used as a means of the social control of women, as in Victorian England. Obviously, *all* of us women in the psychiatric hospital had real problems. I did acknowledge, in my lucid moments, that I did have real difficulties and issues myself and, once I got to know the other women well, they talked about their lives and how they were "being helped to cope". But there was an undoubted element of intervention and control about it all, especially in the way the rebellious patients were treated. Not that I was mutinous at all. I adored Doctor Singh, my consultant psychiatrist. He was so charming, brilliant, beautifully well-mannered, funny and cute. I took to him as soon as I first met him. Even years later, when he left my local outpatients clinic to move on to a bigger and better position, I felt distraught at the thought that I'd probably never see or talk with him again. I felt about him the way I did about Colin, my vicar, that he was a truly good man: it oozed out of every pore of his being. Here was a man devoted to his patients and their well-being: they were his life. You could trust him. He was totally responsible and reliable and would help you, whatever the cost. I miss him like I feel the loss of my vicar, now retired and living in another parish.

The drugs were only one ingredient of my treatment: there was also occupational therapy and the dreaded electroconvulsive therapy: this remedy, horrific, barbaric and terrifying as it was, seemed proof to me, if evidence was needed, of just how ill I was. Only somebody really sick would be prescribed such a horrible, uncivilised therapy, and only somebody so beyond help that they didn't care whether they lived or died would agree to such a savage, drastic procedure. I must have concurred though I really don't remember. I wasn't really well enough to acquiesce or disagree with anything. I didn't trust myself. Even in my murky, sedated state, the thought of such therapy did worry me. It's in my medical notes as a constant refrain that I was worried about the ECT and sought reassurance from the nurses. Doctor Singh explained to me what would happen in simple, scientific words: it sounded appalling, but he did believe it would help me get better and he also pledged that he would always be there to supervise, and I clung to this personal promise like a Titanic survivor clutching on to the side of their lifeboat. I would have a six-week course of ECT treatment, every Monday and Thursday mornings, Doctor Singh decreed. When I was first admitted to the psychiatric hospital, I would have let them cut off my hands and feet, even my arms and legs, if that would have helped me feel better in my head and heart, so desperate and yet, simultaneously, beyond caring did I feel. I knew I had sunk down as far as it was possible to go, so perhaps this extreme measure would help me. Desperate illnesses called for dangerous remedies.

I awoke on Monday 27th of September, the day of my first ECT treatment, gasping for a drink of water as I always did first thing, as the drugs made my mouth so dry. I lurched towards my desk-cum-dressing-table for my bottled water and found nothing! I blinked and stared again. Maybe I wasn't properly awake? I'd had three enormous two-litre bottles of Buxton water that Graham had brought in for me on my table last night. Where had they gone? I questioned my own sanity, once again. Was this something else I was imagining? Or had somebody come in the blackness of the night, while I slept and taken them away? I felt robbed, violated and confused. It was such a strange feeling, on top of all the other "mad" ones. Things always seemed to be disappearing from my room. But who would believe me? Sometimes they appeared again, like my bottled water, which mysteriously reappeared on the Tuesday morning, and sometimes they did not, like my grandmother's marcasite brooch that I used to wear on the lapel of my black jacket. I thought it must have dropped off somewhere, but it was given back to me the day I was discharged. 'We thought you might stab yourself with the long pin clasp,' the duty nurse told me, prosaically. The water had been taken because I wasn't supposed to drink or eat anything, as I was having a general anaesthetic before the ECT treatment.

I was taken with Cynthia, another patient, by a nurse from Mansfield ward to the Byron Day Unit on the same floor, which involved much locking and unlocking of clanging metal doors as I imagine it must sound like in prison. We were then locked in the waiting room alone together, while the nurse went off to see if they were ready for us. In spite of my thick, black depression, waves of fear rippled to the surface of my feelings. The very thought of an electric shock being administered to my brain, strong enough to induce a seizure, like an epileptic fit, seemed so horrific, like some method of ancient diabolical torture. At least, I tried to comfort myself as I paced the waiting room floor, I would be anaesthetised before they blasted me with the electric shock. Doctor Singh had told me that in the past this had not been normal procedure, so patients had experienced the full force of the electric shock and fit themselves. I, at least, should know nothing of it. I would fall asleep and, when I woke up, it would all be over, and I would feel better... surely? But the whole process was very mysterious. Even the all-knowingly God-like Doctor Singh had admitted to me, 'We don't know exactly *how* it works to lift depression, but we do know that it *does* work.'

I wanted to go first to get it over with but the other patient's name was called before mine. I was watching her face very carefully and thought she looked like a French aristocrat ascending to the guillotine, proud and determined to hide her fear. I paced about the waiting room alone and frightened. I thought about running away but knew I was locked in. The only way out was through the treatment room where it was all happening, and I didn't want to go in there at all. I wondered what it was like to watch someone having electric shock treatment and shuddered; because I *did* know: I had seen it once on a television programme. It had traumatised me enough then for me to remember how awful it looked, and now I was about to experience it for myself. Being watched was one of the worst things about it. I was so unusually self-controlled (Doctor Rahman had told me) and a control freak (Doctor Singh himself had called me that!) that I felt sheer, icy horror at the thought of anyone witnessing me lose control and writhe around on the operating table, my arms and legs jerking about, tongue lolling, eyes popping. What if I was to shout or swear or give away my darkest secrets? I felt cold with shame. Eventually it was my turn to be called into the operating room. My heart plummeted when I saw all the people waiting to witness my humiliation. Standing inside were Doctor Singh himself; the nurse who accompanied me; the anaesthetist, obviously; and some other unrecognisable faces. I wanted to scream at them to get out but, of course, could not. There were always one or two youngish, white-coated men present to watch. I know *now* that these were trainee doctors but in my paranoid, disoriented state I'd wondered feverishly if they were people who'd paid to watch the freak show, like those bored, rich people in Victorian London who went to Bethlehem Hospital, known as "Bedlam," to laugh at the crazy antics of the mad people.

I made myself climb up on to the operating table, as bidden, slipping off my glasses. I was glad to take them off as it made all the people goggling at me look all fuzzy and unreal and also, I couldn't see the frightening electrical equipment and rubber paraphernalia. The anaesthetist rubbed a cold gel onto my temples. My black shoes were removed so that they could see my toes twitching, to prove that the current was flowing. I was injected into the back of my left hand and went off into a troubled unconsciousness.

When I came round I felt *frizzled,* as if singed around the edges. Could I smell smoke? I was lying on a trolley and my head ached. The back of my left hand was tender, and I knew it would bruise. I had been warned by Doctor Singh that the ECT would affect my short-term memory, and this was certainly true. I could not remember where I was, why I was there or *who* I was. I looked at my own hands shaking in front of me and didn't know they were mine. My day nurse asked me questions at regular intervals, until gradually my memory came back. She led me back to Mansfield ward and into the dining room where everyone else had just finished breakfast. I had the place to myself, except for the other ECT patient sitting there looking as vacant as I felt, with her nurse. Nobody said a word. My nurse, unusually, served me a breakfast of cornflakes, cold milk, lukewarm toast and hot tea. Normally we inmates helped ourselves, but my hands were shaking so much, I would have dropped anything I managed to pick up. I couldn't even spread the Flora on my toast, so my nurse had to do it for me. They'd given me a muscle relaxant so I didn't break any bones when they induced my fit. It felt like my mind had been rinsed clean. I tried to write in my diary afterwards, but my writing was so wobbly and spidery, like that of an old person, I could hardly make out what I'd written. I couldn't seem to keep many records of what was happening to me: my scrawl was too quivery to read, my memory felt wiped spotless. It was as if they did not want me to know or remember. Or was I being paranoid?

I continued to have regular sessions of ECT treatment until Thursday 7th of October, when the nurses forgot to remove my bottled water from my room and I, thirsty as always, took a long swig of it not knowing what day it was. When the sallow-skinned nurse asked me the routine question of whether I'd eaten or drank anything that treatment day, I had to confess that I'd had some water. This caused tremendous consternation behind the scenes, but I was totally unaware of it at the time, like so much else. I would have to start the whole course of treatment again now I'd missed one, Graham was told, when he rang to inquire how I was. He was very upset, arguing that the ECT be abandoned completely. He didn't like even the thought of it and didn't think it was doing me any good at all. Anyway, I had to have another six sessions, having nine in total.

I imagined that of all the women on the ward, Cynthia, the other ECT patient and I would become friends having shared the intimacy of the procedure together, but we did not. This was partly due to the extreme intensity of our mutual depression and to Cynthia being a smoker. We did our limited socialising in the smoking and non-smoking lounges, respectively. But there was also a palpable feeling that we shared the murky, shameful secret of the ECT treatment that nobody else knew about.

I always preferred to go in first, but the nurses were strictly fair ensuring we took it in turns – one time I'd go in first and the next time, Cynthia. I hated her going first because, left all alone in the waiting room, it was as if I could see what was going on in the treatment room. I couldn't, of course. It would have been impossible. I didn't even go near the light brown door but nevertheless, I could see it so clearly in my mind's eye, I felt like I was watching it on television. I could visualise the table with poor Cynthia stretched out upon it, like a sacrificial victim. The nurse rubbed gel on her temples, before the doctor injected her with a needle in the back of her hand. Another doctor then put a rubber cosh in her mouth, to stop her biting her tongue. Then he buckled a thick, brown strap around her head with two pads on either side of it, like headphones, with lots of wires attached. They must be electrodes. Then, suddenly, they must have administered the electricity because she instantly jerked about, viciously convulsing, throwing out her arms and legs, *writhing* about like a tormented animal caught in a metal trap. Then she shook violently in a tremor down her legs, her arms and all over her twisted body. It was disgustingly, magnetically vivid. I wanted to stop imagining it and drag my thoughts away but everywhere I looked it was *all* I could think about. I felt I was witnessing something I was not meant to. I felt sickened and brutalised and less-than-human, like a shell-shocked soldier in battle, stunned by atrocity and death. And then it was my turn to go over the top. I tried to rearrange my features. Surely, they could see printed on my face what I had just graphically imagined? I lowered my eyes. I wanted to run: but where? I had always felt apprehensive about the ECT treatment but now I could so clearly visualise it to myself, I shrank from putting myself through it. My heart thudding with dread, I forced myself into the room and up on to the table feeling like a tiny atoning lamb led to an enormous ritual slaughter.

When it was over, I reeled up and down my shrinking room, my head aching, as ever, emitting imaginary blue sparks, shaking. I could not stop my quaking and shivering. I felt humiliated; assaulted; abused; shamed; degraded: ripples and waves of all these feelings washed over me. I hadn't done anything wrong. Why were they doing this to me? How long would I be in for? I had no rights, that much was clear to me. I was a scapegoat to be toyed with in a life-or-death game by hospital consultants. I had been persecuted by the baby and now I was being further tortured in this place. They gave me drugs to make me talk and drugs when they wished to keep me quiet, and now, they abused me with electric shocks. I had to get out of this prison; that much was obvious. But how? I was trapped.

After my fit of paranoid delusion, I would sleep. When I woke up, I felt much better like it had all been a bad dream that had happened to somebody else. ECT treatment literally short-circuited the depression in my brain and worked a lot quicker at dispersing it than drugs or therapy.

My mum looked after the baby from Sunday to Friday night and Graham cared for her from Friday to Sunday. This arrangement left him free to visit me every weekday after he'd finished work. My parents (at least my dad, my mum was often too ill) came to see me every Saturday, while my brother Richard and even sometimes John, when he was visiting my parents, came every Sunday. My vicar, Colin came during the day, whenever he could. Not that I always seemed aware that I even *had* visitors, they all apparently complained to each other at the time, which in hindsight seems rather unfair to me, considering how very unwell I was. After my first ECT treatment Graham came to visit, talking to me in the large many-windowed dining room that doubled as the visiting room. I was not allowed to leave Mansfield ward and certainly could not go anywhere on my own, but he asked the nurses for special authorisation to take me out of the confines of the locked ward and for a walk inside the hospital grounds. Graham wanted to ask me, in private, what the ECT treatment had really been like. Permission eventually being granted, I had gone to my room, to fetch my black coat while Graham waited, as visitors were not allowed past the end of the main corridor and in the bedrooms. Half an hour later, I still had not returned and Graham, after sitting alone all this time, feeling abandoned, rejected and anxious, at last told a nurse and she hastened to my room to get me. She found me lying on my bed, staring at the ceiling, having completely forgotten that Graham was there and waiting for me to join him in a walk!

We were let out and tramped out of the main building past the old hospital, which looked soot-blackened and turreted, the very picture of the Victorian workhouse it once was, down a sloping path that led to the ancient, no longer used, pauper's graveyard: a huge field surrounded by threatening greenish black trees. There, in the Autumnal dusk, we walked repeatedly round the outside of the grassland while Graham tried to get me to talk. It was September and he mentioned that faint sniff of chill in the air as we crunched through the red, yellow and brown leaves blown ankle deep, in swirling, drifting piles, the pale sun shining faintly golden as it set. But everything seemed *murky* to me. Heavy, oppressive grey clouds felt like they were fitting closely over my head like a skullcap. And I could not talk because I was aware only of the corpses and the bleached white bones layered upon more corpses and yet more bones, buried and hidden in the ground upon which we walked, grinding them down into ashes and dust. I thought they were groaning yet listening to every word we said. Even in the soft, amber twilight, the place frightened and saddened me. The trees around the outside stood tall, black and stiff like menacing guards around the dead bodies and bones, and we walked around continually, moving on, Graham talking and me silent and terrified. I held my breath and could not speak as twilight fell and darkness came, thinking the bones could hear us and the huge dark green trees were bending forward to listen, closing in on us. Even to reach the pauper's graveyard was scary. We'd had to walk past the two "more secure units" the Dickens and the Shakespeare, both solid, brown-blocked buildings, surrounded by high electric fences. I was intensely preoccupied as to who or what was kept in these "more secure units". I imagined searing cries and petrified screams as I walked past on my way back, searchlights and look-out posts with patrolling dogs and, deep inside, torture chambers. Who were these "criminally insane" people locked away in there? What exactly had they done? Would *I* be next?

Graham didn't think the ECT treatment was doing me any good at all. I seemed to him to be getting worse, not better. My parents and brothers thought the same and I seemed to have stopped thinking and talking altogether. Still, despite Graham's misgivings and protests, the treatment continued and my psychiatrist, at least, told me he was pleased with my progress and if my beloved Doctor Singh was pleased, then so was I.

I was getting so used to the hospital and its routines, I feared I was becoming institutionalised. It was so easy to be told when to get up and what to do. To be given food and told to eat, given tablets and told to sleep. There was no anxiety about going back to work or losing the house, as Graham had told me he feared our house might be repossessed if I didn't go back to teaching. It was all out of my control now. I felt like a tiny child again with no responsibilities. I took my drugs, had my ECT and tried to get better.

I started thinking about the baby again, she was constantly lurking in the depths of my mind. I wondered how she was getting on without her mother. Did I *miss* her? I don't think I did. Graham brought me in a photograph. I placed it on my dressing table to see it all the time. The child looked bigger, older and happier, wearing an unfamiliar bright pink romper suit, her hair flaming like a lit match. Had I damaged her development by this enforced separation? I didn't know. Probably I'd never know. Of course, she was only six months old in September so she wouldn't possibly be able to remember it: or would she? Maybe deep in her psyche somewhere she would be hurt. It was a guilt I would just have to live with, along with all my other mistakes. But surely the child was better off with my parents during the week and Graham at the weekend, with people who loved her and could care for her properly, not me, as I was, then?

My earliest days in hospital are hazy in my memory, as if life was lived under a dim lightbulb. What I most remember is the all-pervading fear that seemed to swirl around me like fog I choked on. Gradually, however, the light seemed to increase, and I became much more aware of everything that was going on both in my head and around me. I noticed how huge, uniformed police officers often appeared on Mansfield ward bringing in some poor woman who had been found babbling to herself, often threatening violence. They were a regular source of excitement to all of us, better than the television.

I used to look around at the sixty-or-so women on my ward and wonder why they were all there. They couldn't all be in for postpartum psychosis, as I was. Many looked far too old to have just had babies. I was curious but I didn't ask, and *nobody* asked me why I was in there. I soon realised that this was the unspoken etiquette of the place, exactly as it probably is in prison. As you gradually got to know people and talked about all sorts of things, the women would tell you odd snippets about their lives and you could surmise from that all you were likely to find out about their particular problem. I'd been born with an open face and a keen ear, and I'd been trained by both my parents to listen to them talk. All my life, old ladies had been telling me their life stories as we waited together in the cold at bus stops, so I was eventually confided in by lots of my fellow patients. I heard harrowing, moving tales of abuse, incest and domestic violence. The women were variously alcoholics; anorexics; bulimics; drug addicts; manic depressives; schizophrenics and even a rumoured attempted murderess. And we were all lumped together on the admissions ward while we were assessed, categorised and then given the treatment we individually needed. The only thing we had in common was that we were all women. All the addictions, compulsions and mental disorders that women could possibly have, we had. But nobody would talk directly about their problems because they were all so ashamed of them. Their "difficulty" had invariably led them to do, or attempt to do, things they regretted immeasurably, and they didn't want to discuss even in privacy with their own psychiatrists. I was just the same: even when talking to the other postnatal depressives (and there were *three* on my ward) I never once admitted that I'd heard voices in my head telling me to *kill* the baby and then myself. Some things just cannot be spoken of; they belong deeply confined in the blackest part of your soul where you dare not venture. They lie in wait for you in your nightmares and make you wake, with a jump, in the small hours, frightened and fighting to breathe as you watch the shadows on the wall, heart thumping.

Some of the inmates were very friendly and seemed "normal". Unfortunately, they were often the ones who had been in for a long time, were at the end of their treatment, "cured" and about to go home. Some women I met only once, others I seemed to see frequently. As I found with Cynthia, the biggest division between the women was among smokers and non-smokers. This was simply because we each had our respective lounges where we could sit in comfortable armchairs and watch television, talk, play bingo and have quizzes. I got to know all my fellow non-smokers. In my entire time in the hospital, I never *once* actually went into the smoking lounge, mainly because it stank of stale cigarette smoke, reeking through the doorway, leaking out into the corridor with that unemptied ashtray stench. The non-smoking lounge seemed larger, perhaps because it usually had less people in it. This seemed a conspicuous design fault of this usually well-designed, newly built hospital. Even to me, hardly an expert, it seemed likely that most of the people with addictive problems: the alcoholics, anorexics, bulimics, drug addicts, and obsessive compulsives would also be smokers, too. (As it happens, I found out that the two lounges were *exactly* the same size, as I had a quick look around when I visited to see the nurses when my daughter started school. It's yet another example of how fear and mental illness can distort the perceptions.) I reasoned to myself that they might have made the smoking lounge smaller to discourage smoking as this was a hospital! But one thing I was not mistaken about was the fact that the smoking lounge, maybe because of its stink and over-crowdedness, always seemed to be in a ferment of discontent, containing louder, more boisterous, more volatile women. The non-smokers certainly seemed quieter, more polite and more approachable to me. All the screaming rows and near fist fights seemed to break out in the smoking lounge or spill out onto the corridor outside, causing the nurses to come running from all directions to calm everyone down with talking, pills and injections.

People often behaved strangely and threateningly, but the only time I saw someone collapse completely and spectacularly was one lunchtime. One pale, thin patient came into the dining room for lunch and fell right over, rigid as an ironing board, hitting the floor with a resonating *thwack*, slamming her head so badly on the corner of the tea trolley that it drew blood. All the nurses panicked badly and flocked to her, dashing at full pelt from every corner of the ward, in an instant. They cleared the dining room at once, so the poor woman could be helped and stitched and I, in my drugged, nebulous state, recalled that I felt miffed I hadn't time to finish my favourite apple crumble! Yet it's in my medical records that I was shaken and upset to see her fall, so I must have told Sarah, the nurse on duty all about it, when I got back to the mother-and-baby unit.

Every inmate had an assigned nurse, our special one, who we could go to for a chat about anything that was bothering us. Mine was called Anne and was lovely and I did tell her a lot, as her records show. Not all the patients were as confiding as me, however. The suspicious Cora used to warn me, "Anything you tell a *screw* (this was how she referred to the nurses) goes straight back to the *governors* (the psychiatrists)." And she was right. I was often surprised at my Friday morning case conference with Doctor Singh when he mentioned something I'd said or done on the ward that he couldn't possibly have witnessed himself. The nurses all watched us constantly and openly made copious notes on everything we patients did or said, even down to where we were at different times of day or night. I was shocked at the level of detail in my hospital records when I received them. Even when I was in bed, I was constantly checked on. The nurses were the eyes and ears (the "grasses" Cora called them) of the all-seeing, all-hearing, all-knowing psychiatrists, the omnipotent gods of the hospital. "Just because you're paranoid," whispered Cora, watching the door, without a flicker of a smile, "Doesn't mean they're *not* out to *get* you."

I moved rooms after about four weeks in the hospital. I was told I *had* to move as someone else needed mine, so two nurses helped me pack my stuff and carry it down the corridor. I hadn't even realised there was a corner with another corridor of rooms beyond it, so fogged in my brain, confined and unadventurous was I then. Paranoid Cora was only in for one day when she was seen covering every square inch of the place. I was being transported further away now I was no longer considered to be high-risk or on suicide watch. They had another emergency patient coming in who needed to be nearer to the nurses. My second room was eerily identical to my first, only being more distant, it took me longer to walk there and back. It also lacked its own clotheshorse on which to spread out my newly washed clothes. This was annoying as it meant that after washing my underwear in the laundry washing machine, I had to leave it spread out on the wooden shelves of the laundry itself, rather than have it dry in the safety of my own room. The laundry was the kleptomaniacs favourite place to filch from, so we all lost several items of clothing; or we just mislaid them, in our befuddled state.

We suffered the ritual of the changing of the bedclothes every Saturday morning on Mansfield. At first, two nurses had helped me with this, as I was correctly deemed to be quite incapable of doing it on my own: it even says so in my medical records. But as I was now judged to be "getting better" I had to do it all on my own: and I *hated* it. First, all the sheets, blankets, covers and pillowcases had to be stripped from my bed and carried, in a huge, awkward bundle to the laundry cupboard. Then I was issued with my clean bedclothes for the week and had to put them back on my bed myself. My murky mental state made it all so confusing. The under sheets had to be the green ones, I think. The over sheets had to be the orange ones and all the pillowcases were pink or was it the other way round? The blankets on top were cream and there was a grey eiderdown on top of the lot, though I could hardly recall it all *then,* never mind *now*. It was so hard to remember where everything was supposed to go. And these were proper old-fashioned sheets and blankets, not the easy, throw-over duvets and covers that I had at home. The nurses came to check later, to ensure that the sheets were smoothed on in the right places and folded neatly into hospital corners. I remember with shame that they always had to redo mine as it was such a pathetic mess. It was like being in the army and being inspected. I would have been sent to the guardhouse every time. How I longed for my own bed and the simple pink floral covers I could throw off with a flick of my wrist. I found it anxiety-inducing and stressful work in my highly sensitive, emotional state and hated Saturday mornings because of it.

    Every evening after supper and dutifully swallowing my drugs, I went, thankfully, to my own room. I knew the nurses locked the office and the whole main section of the ward corridor where the lounges, dining room and laundry were, between about eleven and midnight. I had never been there to see it, as I was obediently trying to get some sleep, but I knew that during the night the nurses camped by the high-risk rooms in tents and sleeping bags because I have very vivid memories of seeing them there, reading magazines under dim green lights and gently leading me back to my room and my bed. I must have been wandering around at night: it says so in my records.

The art studio was a small room just off the main corridor, in which we patients could indulge in creative endeavours. There was a table: paper; paints; assorted coloured card; glue; feathers and sequins. But nobody ever seemed to enter the room for artistic purposes. Nobody ever seemed to make *anything*. After all, there were no scissors in case we stabbed ourselves or each other with them. There was even a record player and some obscurely bizarre vinyl records to play; but nobody ever did.

I was interviewed by Trish, the spiky red-haired occupational therapist in this room and signed up for lots of different classes. There was a huge chart on the wall of the long corridor running down the middle of the ward. It was an enormous whiteboard on which names could be added or erased in coloured markers. I gawped in amazement to see my own name leap out at me, adjoined to the list for virtually every class. (This gigantic whiteboard was *gone* when I went back to visit when my daughter started school, as had the art studio. It was now just a room with seats, filled with four women all fast asleep). Still, I told myself, the classes had to be more interesting than sitting in the non-smoking lounge, trying to knit and having the same conversation as yesterday with my fellow inmates about what we might be having for our tea. I had long ago decided that I would try anything in the hope that it would make me better.

I remember attending some strange classes where we did odd things, such as using the pristine, well-equipped kitchens to make Mars Bar cornflake cakes, for some reason that I never did find out. Maybe it was just meant to be a treat.

I recall a lot of group therapy where we had to sit on our chairs in a big circle and play word association and memory games, such as repeating what the person next to you had told you about themselves. These were usually dull except for the one I most dramatically remember where the therapists all tried to be very optimistic when my friend, an alcoholic, was being urged to tell us about her weekend home leave. The therapists were doing their very best to be cheerful and positive, but a lot of people didn't like taking part either because they were too embarrassed to talk about themselves, too depressed or too dazed on medication to participate. They usually had to coax one of us into saying anything much.

'So, how did your leave go?' one of the therapists asked my friend, once again, smiling brightly.

'Not too well, actually,' she replied, blue eyes downcast, obviously not wanting to talk about it.

'Oh, please share and tell the group all about it,' encouraged another, eagerly.

So, she did. She was reluctant at first but once she'd started, she couldn't seem to stop. 'Well, I was walking home, and I had to go past the pub. I didn't mean to go in but then I thought, I'll just have one and the next thing I knew I was completely *pissed* and refusing to leave at closing time, so they called the police, and I attacked this policewoman, and they arrested me, and I spent the night in the cells on a drunk and disorderly and my sister had to come and bail me out and she brought me straight back here.' Laughter was rare in the hospital, as you would expect, but I'll never forget the horror-stricken looks on the therapists' faces. They desperately tried to put a constructive gloss on it, but this poor woman's tale was just so matter of fact and depressing that they didn't know what to say. I certainly wasn't the only patient there who was dying to laugh out loud at the therapists.

Chapter 9

I loved the MBU

I found most of the occupational therapy baffling so was not sorry when Doctor Singh informed me, at my Friday case conference, that I was now deemed to be so much better that I could move into the mother-and-baby unit at the top of the corridor. I would be there with my child and wouldn't be doing occupational therapy anymore. The MBU was specially cleaned and prepared for me to move into. On the 10th of November 1999 I was helped to relocate permanently into it by two of the nurses. It was a private, self-contained suite consisting of a pink wallpapered sitting room with its own television, two green-painted bedrooms with cots in, an oak-united kitchen and a white-tiled bathroom. It even had its own front door and key, like a separate flat. Its sole drawback was that the big bathroom only had a bath but no shower in it. I preferred a shower for quickness and hygiene's sake. The bath, I was told by the nurses, was in case the new mothers had stitches and so needed to bathe them properly by soaking. (I'd had lots of stitches myself and so thought this very sensible, though I'd never actually personally found the time to have a bath, once the baby was born. However, I still think there should have been a shower, too, as there was enough room and all the other hospital rooms had showers.) The nurses even found and, with cries of joy, unpacked a never-before-used green-checked playpen for my child to sit inside safely and they put it up in the sitting-room.

I loved the MBU and spent all my time in there, though always with at least one nurse present as, "Don't *ever* leave Lorna alone with the baby," had been the rule from the very beginning of my admission. Graham himself had been told this and immediately passed it on to me, thinking it ridiculous. He thought I would *never* harm the child, as did my mum, who was also told never to leave me alone with the baby when I visited her on leave from the hospital. She also ignored their rule, thinking it was nonsense.

I was very worried about being with the baby for most of the time. Graham had brought her in for visits, regularly, after my first few weeks inside. I have a very powerful, distinct memory of watching Graham carrying her in through the door of the ward and up the corridor to me. She was in her car seat carrier and wore a jaunty blue velvet beret on her head and a big pout on her lower lip as she looked around, interestedly.

'Look at that *lip!*' giggled Sharon, the nurse waiting with me, and I felt a huge surge of real anger, my first for ages, at the nurse, for daring to laugh at my precious child. I remember coming forward to greet her, my heart thumping painfully in my chest; and this was just for a short visit in the MBU that had been specially opened for me for the afternoon. Now I was to be with her, and she with me, full time. The only occasions I didn't spend in the MBU were either eating my meals in the dining room or taking the baby out for walks with a nurse.

My new routine once I was in the MBU, was to get up, awakened by the child or a nurse, have a quick bath and get dressed. I would leave to have my breakfast with the other patients in the dining room and then I would return to give the baby her bottle. I would "top and tail" her, washing her face and hands with cotton wool and then change her nappy. Then I would play with her. I would prepare her feeds in the little kitchen, which was where I seemed to spend most of my time: washing bottles; sterilising them; making up feeds and storing them in the fridge. This kitchen was my favourite place in the whole hospital. Not only was it so small that I was virtually left alone and unwatched in there (I revelled in my unusual privacy while the nurses stayed with the baby), but it even had its own tiny window that looked out over the car park in front of the main hospital. This always provided the interesting and ever-changing scene of the real outside world as visitors, doctors and nurses arrived and left. I once saw my beloved Doctor Singh *himself* come out, talking to a group of white-coated men and felt elated, like I'd had a private glimpse of royalty.

But the thing I liked best and really enjoyed was to take the baby out in the pram with Enid, my favourite nurse. The child would be wrapped in her own blankets but strapped into the hospital's own pram. I remember the first time we took her outside I was pushing the pram and found it really difficult. Typically, I thought it was me being weak and pathetic, so I struggled along, straining and shoving. After *miles* I told Enid I felt exhausted, so she went to push the pram and the moment she did, she said, "Oh, you've left the brake on! No wonder you found it hard to push." We would walk around the diminutive, picturesque village and look in the few shops and at the chocolate-box cottages. "Outside" seemed enormously huge to me, after being confined in hospital rooms for so long. The sky seemed so far away and miraculously always changing. The whole world seemed magically to come *alive* for me, all brightness and busyness and I came alive too, along with it. I loved going out. It made me feel "normal" again and it was such a relief to have escaped the oppressive atmosphere of the volatile ward and to be out in the open and in soothing nature, breathing proper invigorating air again, even though the weather was rather cold. It was November and frosty, so even though we bundled ourselves up warm, our skin tingled and glowed pink. These trips out with my motherly nurse, Enid, looking at ordinary things but through newly opened eyes, talking about everyday matters with a rekindled interest were the best therapy I received from the hospital in my whole stay. At last, I began to realise the possibility of a life outside the hospital, a good, regular existence that I could have with my baby and my husband, in which everything would be fine, once more. I clung onto this hope like a shipwrecked sailor clambering on top of wreckage, desperate to survive.

Joanne, one of the nurses, labelled all my baby equipment in the kitchen with "Natalie" stickers. When I asked why, she said there was another mother coming into the MBU with her daughter, so it was to stop her using any of my child's things. This fussy nurse was the only one who asked me a very tricky question.

'Why don't you pick her up and give her a cuddle?' she said one day when the child was fretting and we were alone.

'I don't believe in picking children up every five minutes and spoiling them,' I told her sternly, my heart pounding. I sounded like my mum. Joanne just turned away to reach for another toy, but I knew I had been found out. The truth was, I was *still frightened* of the baby. Even now I regarded her as something of an undischarged missile in my life. I found my daughter's presence so anxiously troubling; I wondered if I would ever get used to her.

I was glad to be mainly off the ward as it was a very temperamental place. The notice on the doors that could be read outside stated boldly, "Due to the volatile nature of the ward, these doors must remain locked." (When I went back to visit, this notice had gone and was replaced by a bell to ring and a staffed reception desk near the door, to let people in and out.)

Most women were subdued when they arrived on the ward and, if not, were very soon sedated into submission, but not Cora. Despite the massive amount of medication she was prescribed, Cora was still extremely astute and explosive. I had witnessed her being issued with drugs and heard her argue about *every single tablet,* though maybe she didn't swallow them? I supposed it could be done, though with great difficulty. On her very first day on Mansfield, she nearly started a fight and the whole thing was witnessed by Graham. He was walking up the corridor on his way to see me in the MBU, when he passed the payphones by the door of the non-smoking lounge. Cora was yelling to harangue some hapless person on the phone and Sylvia was standing next to her, purse in hand, obviously waiting to use the phone but positioned very close and gawping.

'What the *fuck* are you staring at?' Cora screamed at her, mid-tirade, baring her perfect white teeth.

Graham was now used to Sylvia's strange yet harmless ways but thought the newly arrived and dangerously turbulent Cora was about to *hit* her, so reckoned he'd better intervene.

'She's only waiting to use the phone,' he told Cora, helpfully.

'I'm only waiting to use the phone,' echoed Sylvia, peaceably.

'Well, YOU can fuck off,' began Cora, pointing an aggressive forefinger in her direction, 'And so can YOU!' She discharged her lethal forefinger at Graham and then turned to face him, belligerently, as if she might lash out. A vigilant nurse was watching, as usual, and she came out to tell Cora to calm down, so the poor nurse received the full impact of her angry outburst and both Graham and Sylvia were free to walk away. He arrived, flustered in the

MBU and told the nurse and me all about it. Cora and Sylvia became unlikely friends, as it happened. I witnessed it myself, the next day, in the dining room. Cora was sitting on her own, glowering to herself when Sylvia sat right next to her, as closely as she possibly could.

'What the *fuck* do you want from me?' Cora yelled at her.

Sylvia smiled adoringly at her and rested her head on Cora's shoulder. 'I just want you to *love* me,' she said, so sweetly and innocently that even Cora laughed and put her arm around her, and they were inseparable after that.

Graham was appalled at the news that another psychiatrist, (not my Doctor Singh, of course) wanted to move one of his patients into the MBU with her baby. He argued with everybody, all the nurses and even with the other patient's psychiatrist and Doctor Singh himself, secretly, without being obvious, trying to prevent the other mother from moving into the MBU, saying it would set back *my* recovery irretrievably.

He managed to postpone it for a week but Sue, the other mother, did move in and changed things a great deal. Instead of lounging in the sitting room, we had to stay in my bedroom to play with the baby while Sue stayed in her bedroom with her child.

Cora remained the most interesting inmate. She had all her faculties sharpened and ready to stab when everyone else kept calm and mellow.

'The word hysteria comes from the Latin for womb,' she informed me one day, over lunch. She was right. I had an A-level in Latin. 'And always remember, all men think all women are mad anyway, and all the psychiatrists in here are *men*.' I knew she had a valid point. I'd felt before that they seemed to want to cure us of being women and make us more like men.

One day, when I was passing on my way to take the baby out for a walk with Enid, pushing the blue pram, I witnessed Cora publicly ranting and yelling offensively at her psychiatrist as she pursued him all the way down the corridor, until the unhappy man escaped out of the ward doors, hurriedly unlocked by a nurse. Cora tried to follow him and had to be restrained by two nurses, to stop her. They told her to calm down and offered her a sedative, but Cora would not be cowed.

'Fucking screws, that's all you are!' she shouted at them and lashed out. There were immediately two other nurses there and they dragged Cora off into a side room.

'What'll happen to Cora?' I gasped, horrified. I *knew* she had gone too far this time.

'They'll take her to a more secure unit,' Enid told me.

'The rubber room in Colditz?' I asked, petrified. I had listened to horrific rumours about this place and walked past it often on my walks outside. All the inmates had heard shocking stories of what went on inside and delighted in spreading them around.

'They're called the Dickens or the Shakespeare units,' Enid told me, reassuringly. 'She'll get the help she needs. Now, don't you go worrying about her, she's brought this on herself.' But I couldn't help feeling anxious about her; and torn. I couldn't decide what to do or even whether I could do anything at all. I did guiltily admire Cora and her rebellious attitude and intelligence, while deploring the way she behaved.

I never saw Cora again. And I never did find out what happened to her. She just seemed to *disappear*. I asked all the nurses, but they just said she'd been moved somewhere more secure and that was that. It was whispered hysterically on the ward that she'd been dragged off screaming, swearing and kicking in a straitjacket to have a lobotomy; but that was just the fear talking: I hope.

The only person in the entire hospital more stubborn and argumentative than Cora was turning out to be my normally mild-tempered husband. He really was my hero, fighting for me all the time, as I was in no fit state to do it myself. I didn't realise then how much he was doing behind the scenes, having meetings and conferences and phone calls with lots of different staff when I wasn't there. It's all written in my medical records, as a constant chorus, "The patient's husband complained..." crops up repeatedly. He wanted the ECT stopped; he wanted my medication changed; he wanted me in the MBU; he didn't want another mother and baby in the MBU with me; he wanted me on leave; he wanted me discharged. I was amazed and delighted when I finally realised how much he had been battling for me.

I only asked for my medical records years later, knowing how upset I'd be looking at them. I often felt like I was reading about something that had happened to someone else. The doctors and nurses' comments go on repetitively and yet I have no memory of a great deal of it; even the more embarrassing incidents such as wetting myself at night. You'd think the shame alone would have imprinted this on to my mind but no. I felt shocked and humiliated when I read the nurses' reports. And there was another dreadful night when I was told to put on my nightdress, which I just stared at for hours, before finally putting it on *over* my clothes. A nurse had to help me undress, put it on properly and get back into bed. I'm also described as aimlessly wandering the corridors, laughing inappropriately to myself, repeating everything that was said to me and not making any sense. I don't remember *any* of this and am thankful that I don't. To add to all these incidents that I don't recall, I have several episodes that I remember very vividly yet they do *not* appear in my notes at all.

Another very odd thing about reading my medical records is that they're all about me. Hardly anyone else is mentioned, except for the baby, an inmate of the MBU and, of course, Graham, who is referred to nearly as often as me but never by name. He is written as "the patient's husband," constantly complaining, indicating how worried he was about me and the child. The other patients are never named and only alluded to in passing. I'm described as upset and anxious in the early days because some inmates have told me that I'll have my baby taken off me, put into care and will never get her back! Often the mood on the ward is stated to be volatile, but these are all fleeting references. What I *mainly* remember when I think about being in the psychiatric hospital are the other inmates milling round, talking or silent, acting strangely, threateningly or pleasantly. The patients made a much stronger impression on me than the doctors or nurses, probably because they were more interesting due to being less inhibited, restrained and busy. Yet they are strangely absent from my medical records. Reading them, it's as if I had the whole place virtually to myself.

It was very weird to see the number of meticulous notes kept on my behaviour, progress, tests, medication and how I was with the baby on an hourly basis. It's very odd to have been so closely observed and to have been so disorientated that I didn't even notice, as I'm normally very self-conscious and aware when I'm being watched. It is a tearful experience to see a part of your life set out before you in cold, clinical notes, that you remember so little about; it is like a black hole where your memories should be. But I am so grateful for these copious records: they have certainly helped me fill in the gaps and I'm so thankful to have them, however strange and painful they are to read.

I remember my hands shaking very badly so I was given Procyclidine for drug side effects rather than anxiety. This is given to people with Parkinson's disease to stop trembling, and is often given to psychiatric patients who are experiencing shaking because of the antipsychotic drugs. I was quivering all over and pacing around repeatedly at that time. I remember my brother Richard coming to visit, without John, and I complained to him about John walking about continually and not sitting still. I'll never forget the sad look he gave me. '*Someone* was pacing up and down all the time,' he told me, "But it wasn't John, and it wasn't me.' I recall the deep shame I felt.

On the 28th of October it was my 40th birthday and I had my 9th and final ECT. Apparently two of the nurses saw in my records that it was my birthday, and I was forty, so they woke me up singing, 'Happy Birthday to you'. Shamefully, when I awakened, I told them it *wasn't* my birthday, and I certainly was not forty! They told me this when I was officially discharged on the 10th of December, and I felt really embarrassed as I couldn't remember this at all. Still, at least it set me up for a lifetime of winning the "How miserably I spent my fortieth birthday" game, often played at parties. I still have never met anyone who can top, "I spent my fortieth incarcerated in a lunatic asylum having electric shock treatment!"

I was moved into the mother-and-baby unit on Wednesday the 10th of November, and I was in such a dreadful state of anxiety that I couldn't settle for one minute without shaking all over and having to *pace* around. The nurse noted that I fed the baby at midnight and told her I was "being tortured" because the child was crying. I was described as "anxious and very tired." The baby slept from 1:15 a.m. but I could not relax. I was complaining of rigidity in my arms. I was given diazepam and slept from 3:15 a.m. onwards. In the morning I was very nervous when dealing with the baby. I was sweating profusely and extremely shaky. I told the nurse I was frightened in case I hurt the baby when I was doing things for her. I was still perspiring and anxious when tending to the child in the evening.

That night, on the 11th of November, I woke at 1 a.m. expressing extreme anxiety. I tried to rest but could not. I was given Valium and sleeping pills, but they didn't work. I was walking up and down in my room until staff "strongly advised" me to lie down. I do remember this very well. It was the most *agitated* I've ever been in my life. I wanted to relax but simply could not. My mind and body would not let me. I told the nurse I felt anxious, couldn't cope and wanted to harm myself, bang my head against the wall and end it all. I told the nurse that the baby had to leave the unit until I'd recovered and that I had been hiding my feelings. I was sweating profusely, unable to sit down and felt nauseous. The nurse noted that I continued like this without sleep until 6 a.m. I felt like one of the walking dead. The whole night was one long torturous panic attack, and I couldn't settle for one moment. I *shook* all over as soon as I lay down feeling like an alien might emerge from my stomach and attack me. It was the presence of the baby that upset me so much. I still regarded her as an undetonated missile that could explode at any second. But the nurses were absolutely right when they told me the longer I cared for the baby, the more we would get used to each other and bond. My time in the mother-and-baby unit was absolutely invaluable because every day we bonded more and more so when I was finally discharged on the 10th of December, I had a good idea of how to cope.

Chapter 10

Recovery

It shocks me in my medical records to see all the numerous drugs I was given. At first I was put on Cipramil, an antidepressant, and later Paroxetine, another antidepressant, to treat depression, anxiety and panic attacks. I was also given Stelazine, an antipsychotic tranquilliser used in higher doses to treat schizophrenia and related conditions, very bad agitation or dangerous behaviour. I was also prescribed Procyclidine, an anticholinergic medicine used to treat Parkinsonism resulting from treatment with antipsychotic drugs. I insisted I was issued with a contraceptive pill too, terrified that I would get pregnant again and suffer more postpartum psychosis (even though I wasn't having sex!). I was also given Diazepam (Valium), an anti-anxiety drug and muscle relaxant, which also helps treat anxiety related insomnia. Moreover, I was given Stilnoct, a sleeping drug and Melleril, yet another antipsychotic tranquilliser. Once I'd left hospital I was also prescribed lithium carbonate, used to treat with antidepressants, more resistant depression and to stabilize my moods.

At some time before my discharge meeting something very strange and wonderful happened: I felt like I was given back my real beloved Natalie. She was the beautiful girl born in the maternity hospital and I'd adored her right from the start, having a mystical experience of unconditional love when I was breastfeeding her. But something went terribly wrong. She changed into a *demon child* and started torturing and persecuting me. She became "it"; "the baby"; "the child"; not my beloved Natalie at all. Somehow the psychiatric hospital gave *her* back to me. I was so happy to have her back, so relieved and joyful.

I was discharged on the 10th of December 1999, and Natalie's very first Christmas, looked forward to with so much anticipation, was, of course, an anti-climax. I was still in a highly nervous state. I'd had very little time for shopping, so had just three small toys for her. I'd wanted to buy her a whole toy shop of her own, but Graham reminded me that Natalie was only nine months old, didn't know what Christmas was, nor would she remember it, though I took lots of photographs, so that she could look back on it and see how much we loved her.

On Christmas morning, all sat around our twinkling lighted Christmas tree, we opened Natalie's few presents: a street scene of red houses that lit up and played tunes when you pressed brightly coloured buttons; a Teletubby toy; and a blue sorting cube that took different shapes in through various spaces. She loved fiddling about with them all. Graham had bought me three lovely presents: an Opium gift set; Thornton's continental chocolates; and a compact disc of 60's and 70's classic hits (though The Supremes' *Baby Love* wasn't on it, I'm glad to say). I was surprised because Christmas for me now was all about Natalie, not us. I'd only bought one present for Graham. It was a blue shirt, and he was delighted with it, even though it was hardly a surprise as he'd been with me in Marks & Spencer when I bought it, Natalie cradled to his chest as he pretended to look the other way. We had Christmas dinner at my parents', and I tried to get into the Christmas spirit and relax even though I wasn't allowed to drink alcohol because of taking antidepressants and lithium. I also *had* to keep obsessively checking on Natalie when she fell asleep, to make sure she was still breathing and all right. Despite all this, we got through it.

In 1999 the Prime Minister was Tony Blair. His Labour Government had swept to power in a landslide victory in 1997. The NHS seemed to me to be working very well because it appeared properly funded. It seemed very easy for me to see doctors as and when I needed them, and as soon as I required it, I got my place in the newish, purpose-built psychiatric hospital with the wonderful mother-and-baby unit, which was very well-staffed with numerous health workers. I think I was very lucky and got marvellous treatment that saved mine and my baby's life. The NHS aftercare was also very good. After Christmas I was visited every weekday morning by the community psychiatric nurse from the local mental health clinic. Doctor Singh had introduced me to Michelle at my discharge meeting and I had liked her immediately, with her kind blue eyes and lop-sided smile. She had asked me what time of day she should come round to see me and Natalie, and I had requested that she come at ten every morning. I'd chosen that time deliberately so I wasn't tempted to stay in bed or sit around in my dressing gown. I would have to get up, shower and dress myself and Natalie before she arrived. Michelle's visits gave shape to my day, but it was also rather bad timing because Teletubbies came on television then and Natalie and I *loved* it. It was absolutely our favourite programme, the only show that I could watch with completely unadulterated happiness. I am not ashamed to say I found it wonderfully soothing as it consisted of fresh green fields, bright red and yellow flowers and silly, harmless creatures having fun, talking baby language that both Natalie and I understood perfectly. Nothing *bad* ever happened in Teletubby land and this was exactly what I wanted and needed in my own little kingdom. So, while Michelle talked, Natalie and I furtively watched the calming Teletubby images on the screen, with the sound turned down. Their presence made me feel better, though I was rather frustrated that I couldn't have the volume up and view it properly. Still, Michelle was an engaging, helpful woman and Natalie and I both liked her very much. It was the new Millenium and the whole world seemed to be celebrating a new start and so was I.

I had appointments to see Doctor Singh once every fortnight for three months, then every month for six months, and after that every two months. I then saw one of his team of psychiatrists and psychologists (sometimes the lovely and familiar Doctor Rahman) every three months rather than Doctor Singh himself. I missed talking with him, of course, but it was my own fault: I was getting better. The other psychiatrists and psychologists were all pleasant and attentive men. We had interesting discussions about how dreadful the first year with a new baby could be and whether postnatal depression really *was* a mental illness or not as it was so widespread amongst mothers, to some degree.

After one whole year Doctor Singh decided that I didn't need a community psychiatric nurse to visit me anymore. Michelle had been superseded by the charming Annie and her visits had dwindled to just once a week, so I was quite used to a nurse not coming. Natalie and I were starting to get on with our lives without them. After two years Doctor Singh decided I didn't need to see any more health professionals and I was completely discharged from the clinic into the care of my local doctor's surgery. I felt sad that I wouldn't see my beloved Doctor Singh again but realised, with a shock, that I really didn't need him or any of his team anymore.

One of the best things Michelle advised me to do was to attend a regular, local mother-and-toddler group. There was one at my nearby church's annexe, so we went to that every Wednesday afternoon and it was perfect for getting us out of the house and mixing with other mothers, babies and children. I made more friends there than I had in ten years of living in the village and our children went to the local church school together.

Not everything was that simple, however. A woman I met in psychiatric hospital lived quite near to me. Once I was released, I'd walk past her house often, drawn to it against my will. On the neat row of terraces, hers was the only house with chipped, discoloured paintwork and dirty windows, where the faded green curtains were always closed. *I* felt like that house sometimes: down at heel, sad, withdrawn, seemingly empty. Every time I walked past pushing my golden-haired daughter in her blue pram, I expected her to come out and point at me, stinking of foul-smelling drugs, hair wildly loose, face crazed, identifying me as a fellow madwoman. It never happened yet I lived in terror of it, every single day.

On the 26th of September, Natalie had her eighteen-month check up by the health visitor who said she was very far ahead of where she should be, which made me relieved. Perhaps I hadn't damaged her development as much as I feared.

Being completely discharged by the clinic and getting better had taken a lot longer than I had expected. But I could joke with Graham about it now. 'I've gone from being *psychotic* to being merely *neurotic* again, so that's practically cured,' I told him.

I loved Natalie more than my own life and could hardly believe that there had ever been a time when this was not so. I was constantly surprised at the overwhelming intensity and passion of my relationship with my daughter. I loved her totally and unconditionally. Nobody could upset me more than Natalie, but nobody could delight me more and make me feel that blessed, universal, unqualified love.

For all the mad and bad thoughts, the fact remains that I never actually *did* what those terrible voices in my head told me to do. I never harmed one golden hair on her perfect little head: not once, not *ever,* though the voices were bombarding me with evil suggestions, all the time. The only occasions I had to take her to the doctor's surgery were for her immunisation injections, nappy rash and some tiny bleeding after her umbilical cord fell off. The only time I ever had to take her to A&E was when she'd started school and developed a water infection because she was too frightened to ask to use the toilet in school. I've never hit or smacked her, which is an achievement when you consider I was continually hit as a child, by my mum, my dad *and* my older brother.

We went on our first family holiday together to the Isle of Man. I remember feeling surprised by how genuinely happy I felt once more at being with Natalie and Graham. We walked on the beach at Douglas, just across the road from our hotel. We strolled by the gently lapping sea and paddled together in the rock pools. I had never felt so joyful in my entire life. The drugs had kept me from feeling desperately depressed, but they had also taken away my highs with my lows. They kept all my emotions steadily fixed, like a straight line on a graph but I missed my happy peaks. Now, with my doctor's advice, I was coming off the antidepressants and the lithium, slowly, gradually cutting down on the dosages. By December I would be completely drug-free but already I was feeling the benefits. On lithium and the antidepressants, I felt nothing: it was like being dead, a robot going through the motions of a life, not really feeling it. I missed my strong emotions desperately, so coming off the drugs was like coming back to life. My world changed from grey to glorious technicolour. I loved having my intense emotions back: even the negative ones were better than feeling numb, indifferent and barely alive. I felt bored when I wasn't strongly aroused and passionate about my life. I was used to extremes because of my past. I could handle it all now.

    I looked out at the glorious endless view and felt completely *suffused* with happiness. A golden light seemed to leap and dance on the rippling sea. The foam frothed like cream on the edge of the squelching sand. The brilliant white seagulls wheeled in the air before resting for a few moments on a shifting, glistening sandbank. They faced the same way, watching the sun glittering on the wet sand, taking wing as one bird, curving their fluttering path against the dazzling sun, touching the turquoise, sparkling sky. The blonde beach was one enormous, undulating curve, bordered by the massively stretched sea. Green rock pools teemed with life; strange transparent creatures flicked and wriggled through the water. Trickling currents were diverted around curling, twisted shells. We heard the constant calling of the seagulls, smelt the sea salt in the air, saw the mist surging in over the hills, heard the crash of the wind, of waves smashing on the rocks, saw the iridescence of green and pale blue pools inside the darker blue of the sea water.

    I felt as if transported out of myself in joy and saw my own happiness reflected upon me in the faces of Natalie and Graham. All these perfect moments I'd had in my life were like beads on a mala or rosary I could finger on my deathbed, saying, "I have lived. I have known real joy, genuine bliss, true love". I felt fully suffused with satisfaction, truly loved and blissfully content. These were the moments I thought of and treasured, the ones I would always have, not too frequent to be commonplace, not too infrequent to be mythical but enough to show it was possible to be euphorically happy in my life, in spite of pain, grief and loss. At these moments I throbbed with vitality, as a component of everything around me: I was in it and it was in me, all part of the whole pattern that the universe was constantly weaving, making everything *new*. It was then that I knew everything was connected. Everything was connected to me, and I was connected to everything else. Time stood still.

Everything in my life seemed to have led me to this moment. I wanted to say, 'I'll never be unhappy again,' although I knew I would be, but I also knew that I'd still be all right. I would cope. I was strong. I had broken and been shattered into miniscule fragments, but I had put myself back together with lots of help, assembling myself piece by tiny piece until I knew I was whole again. I knew I'd always be blessed with this knowledgeable love I had, and felt that I'd always be aware of it hovering around me, even in the worst times. There would inevitably be bad times, but it would still be there, waiting for me to reach it again. I smiled at Graham beside me and at my daughter, Natalie. Clutching my beloved child, I knew I never could and never would let her go again and I was glad, happy and content, *at last*.

But even though I felt so much better I still didn't know why my life had gone so catastrophically wrong, and I'd ended up going mad and confined to psychiatric hospital. I knew I needed to explore my past.

Chapter 11

Trying for a baby

When I married Graham in July 1989 he was as keen to start a family as I was and so we started trying for a baby. I couldn't believe it when I didn't get pregnant right away. And all around me, of course, everyone was having babies. *Everywhere* I looked, all I could see were pregnant women and children. My mum was obviously wondering why Graham and I had not yet produced the requisite grandchild and, typically for her, didn't ask directly, just chose to tell us continually and obsessively how everybody else in the entire world was having babies except us. It *ruined* our Christmases for ten miserably dragging years. We always thought: why can everybody else have babies and not us? The very worst thing about teaching children was that the parents were constantly producing more babies. It was like a conveyor belt, and they were always brought to me, at the insistence of the child in my class. I then had to coo over and cuddle them as if I wasn't desperately envious. I also knew, naturally, several families in which children were being neglected or abused. It was all so unfair. What had Graham and I done to deserve this? All we wanted was *one* baby of our own.

I told Graham that something must be medically wrong either with me or him or, god forbid, both of us and so began our convoluted round of doctors, examinations, tests and referrals to hospitals and specialists. I'm not criticising the NHS or any of the hospitals and specialists we consulted. I'm sure all the correct procedures were followed as quickly as possible, but it all took up so much TIME and I felt my fertility ebbing away by the day. With each month that passed it was like I was losing the chance to have the baby we so desperately wanted and needed. I had a laparoscopy and hysterosalpingography to check that my fallopian tubes were open, and they were. Finally, we were referred for IVF just as we were simultaneously trying to sell our first house.

Graham was undergoing his own separate round of tests and referrals. Consulting one urologist at his top floor clinic on a row of posh houses, he'd taken off his clothes so the man could examine him physically. This was embarrassing enough and uncomfortable as the urologist grabbed his genitals very hard, feeling for any lumps or irregularities. Then Graham happened to glance up out of the window and saw the whole top deck of a passing green bus which was packed with elderly ladies in hats, staring down at them, looking shocked and disgusted!

We found a new house and moved in delightedly, telling each other, "New house, new baby!"

We seemed to wait months for hospital appointments which were just for quick, simple blood tests. It all took up so much time, exactly what we most lacked. I was now thirty-three, described by doctors to my face as "elderly" to be trying for a first baby. Quietly but relentlessly we could see our chances of having a healthy child escaping from us; my monthly eggs felt like grains of merciless sand spilling through an egg-timer.

My body became my enemy. I was examined so much I felt like a lump of meat on a butcher's slab and what was even worse, a defective, useless hunk of carcass. "Unexplained infertility" was stamped ineffaceably on my medical file and, I felt, on my very soul. Two different doctors had told us that we seemed unlikely to have a child of our own and encouraged us to adopt. It just made me more furiously determined. I didn't *care* what the medical specialists said: I WAS going to have a baby. I was becoming absolutely obsessed. From my first conscious thought on waking to the last solid idea in my head at night, all I could think about was having a child. But the waiting list for IVF at the NHS hospital was *five years!*

'We'll have to go private,' I told Graham. He agreed. We knew it would be expensive, but we would find the money somehow. The private clinic's front garden was dominated by an enormous apple tree. I watched entranced as the faint breeze blew the pink and white blossoms down from the dark branches, so that it looked like it was snowing. As we walked hesitantly up the front path, petals lay strewn beneath us in a scented carpet fit for a princess in a fairy tale. I felt sure this was an enchanted place where magical miracles happened.

Doctor Cohen, the eminent gynaecologist who interviewed us, sat behind his huge mahogany desk in his wood-panelled office and told us how expensive it would be and, much worse, he told me to *lose weight* before I started IVF. In just over four months I lost two stone in weight, despite working full-time as a teacher. I didn't go to any slimming clubs or follow any special diet plan. I just went about it in the simplest and hardest way: I ate a lot less and I exercised a lot more. It was *really hard.* I was exhausted and stressed but I did it. From when I was young, food had been my great comfort and mainstay, my way of coping with tiredness and pressure. I've never smoked or taken drugs and barely drank alcohol: food was all I needed and now I couldn't have that. Every single crumb I put in my mouth, I asked myself, "Is this helping me or hindering me from having a baby?" Every bite or sip was psychologically monitored, and it worked. I lost twenty-eight pounds in just over four months because I wanted a child more than I wanted or needed food. Nothing was more important: it dominated absolutely every waking second of my life.

It called to mind my father's favourite dietary advice to me, repeated often throughout my tender, sensitive teenage years, 'If you want to lose seven pounds of ugly fat just cut off your head!' Then he'd guffaw away to himself at my hurt face. My brother John sniggered away too. They both thought this hilarious. *I didn't.*

Mum was no help, 'If you want to lose weight, just bloody *move! Do some housework!*' was her constant mantra, as she puffed away on a cigarette.

The IVF procedure was always the same, simultaneously incredibly boring yet intensely stressful. After a long drive filled with nauseous tension in nerve-wracking traffic, I'd then wait to see the sombre-faced radiographer who would scan my ovaries using a vaginal probe. I had to lie back on the couch while she eased the probe into me and then checked the monitor for results. I would then wait to see the nurses who gave us needles and syringes. Later in the afternoon, I'd have to phone the surgery once a doctor had seen my report. Then I'd be told I could start the Buserelin injections. (I'd ordered the drugs on Doctor Cohen's prescription, through our local chemist.)

I'd dash home from school, driving as fast as I dared. Sitting in front of my dressing table I'd attach a needle to a syringe with quivering fingers, as I'd been shown by the nurses. (I *hated* needles and always had but realised it was yet another phobia I'd have to conquer to get the baby I so desired.) I stuck the syringe into the top of the phial of Buserelin and pulled the needle until it sucked up the exact amount I needed: 0.5 millilitres. Next, I had to flick the syringe with the nail of my middle finger, to make sure there were no air bubbles in it. I squeezed the flesh at the top of my thigh into a roll of flab, before taking a deep breath, *stabbing* the needle into it and then plunging the syringe down. Of course, it stung and left a bruise. I had to do this daily with a fresh needle and syringe, until the clinic told me to stop. Every day it hurt, especially when I accidentally injected into an old bruise: that made me wince with pain.

It was long, arduous and both physically and mentally draining. And for someone of my temperament – anxious, driven, impatient, emotionally volatile – who liked to be in control of what was happening to me and around me, it was *extra* difficult. Plus, I was teaching full-time, and I found it a very stressful job.

The Buserelin acted to downregulate my ovaries. The symptoms were like the menopause. Typically, I experienced them *all:* irritability; tiredness; headaches; anxiety; hot flushes and night sweats.

Everyone around me, even my teaching colleagues, seemed constantly to be having children. Everywhere I looked all I seemed to see were tanned, happy women pushing bright-eyed babies in immaculate, frilly-lined prams. 'They look like tarts pushing their knickers around,' I'd comment, acidly, to Graham.

The worst thing about my fellow workers getting pregnant was that nobody ever told me. Everyone else in the whole school knew for ages before the headteacher found the courage to break the news to me. I felt like an outcast, forced to walk around ringing a bell, croaking, "Barren! Infertile! Not a real woman!"

All this time, Graham and I were regularly visiting John in hospital in London. It was an incredibly stressful time. It nearly *destroyed* me. My legs were a muddled mess of violet, purple and yellow splodges and were achingly sore from the Buserelin injections. I couldn't touch or rest my hands on them for even one second because they felt like tender, pulverised meat. Once, in the early days, I forgot and crossed my legs. I nearly passed out from the pain. I didn't do *that* again.

About the thirty-first day of my cycle, I'd bleed. Then I'd have another scan to make sure I was ready to start the

FSH injections: more waiting around to be seen. The sonographer would check with a vaginal probe to see that my ovaries were downregulated. I'd have to phone later to check I could start the FSH injections; these would stimulate my ovaries into producing a lot of eggs rather than just the usual one for the month. I also had to continue to inject myself with the Buserelin daily so that my normal cycle didn't intervene to disrupt the treatment. This ensured that the FSH was in control of my cycle and could work unimpeded. Once I had the permission to proceed, I would go to the doctor to start the Pergonal 75IU (two lots of the stuff). He was a sweet man, but he struggled somewhat. Later, I found out at my clinic when *they* did it, that he was supposed to have snapped the drug ampoule in two to open it, instead of unorthodoxly *beating* it with metal tongs over a wastepaper bin! (What did the other patients in the waiting room think of the violent din?) The Pergonal had to be injected into the muscles of my bottom which was why I couldn't do it myself. After one week on the Pergonal I had hot flushes, headaches and stomach pains. Then I needed another scan. The sonographer told me how many follicles were growing in each ovary. Not every follicle would produce an egg, however. Soon my ovaries would feel rather swollen and tender, like over-ripe plums about to burst. Then I'd need daily blood tests to make sure my ovaries were not hyperstimulated as they could rupture, and this could lead to death. Then there was the increased risk of ovarian cancer that all women having fertility treatment faced. I could be literally *dying* to have a child.

This stage was so *painful*. I'd often wake and immediately double up in excruciating pain and in desperate need to go to the toilet. This agony was caused by my full bladder pressing on one of my swollen ovaries. I'd often feel nauseous and want to vomit. I'd usually lie on the bathroom floor feeling sick and dizzy until it eventually passed, and I started to feel better. At the next scan the sonographer could measure the size of the follicles in my ovaries. She gave me a notepad and pencil and I'd jot down the figures she'd call out to me.

When the follicles were big enough, we'd be on "The Midnight Run," going back to the main private hospital at midnight to have the hCG injection that would trigger ovulation. Then, thirty-six hours later, I'd be going into hospital for the egg recovery.

This was the very worst part. I'd be taken from my private room, bundled onto a wheeled trolley by two male porters, pushed into the lift and taken up to the operating theatre on the third floor. The dazzlingly white searching lights in the lift and in the operating theatre hurt my sensitive eyes. I always felt nervous and very alone waiting to go in, though the nurses would try chatting to me.

The anaesthetic needle always looked and felt huge, surely too big to be jabbed into the thin, blue vein protruding on the back of my left hand. It felt like a sharp dagger being plunged in. I *hated* the next part where they slipped the rubber mask over my nose and mouth. My survival instinct always made me want to drag it off but instead I forced myself to take long, deep breaths. I wanted to get on with it and go under quickly. The anaesthetist's voice would sound far away saying, 'Just giving you a little oxygen now,' and I'd smell this extra-fresh seaside air that tasted cool and pure, but it soon changed within seconds to the murky, smoky gush of the gas. This was horrible: then came the blurring of faces, like they were wax dummies melting and the slowing down and slurring of voices into hazy, indistinct, un-tuned radio sounds. Swiftly following this came the repetitive "duh duh duh" noise, like bass notes going down a musical scale, followed by a sudden high-pitched "Ping! DUH duh duh duh Ping!" On and on it went…

When I slowly became aware of things again, I'd find myself laid out on a trolley once more, nobody near me. That first time I'd felt something squeezing hard on the top of my left arm: I panicked! Was I having a heart attack? Then it stopped tightening and released itself. I turned my head, groggily, to look in its direction. It was a machine compressing my arm in a steel armband. I realised it must be some sort of automatic blood pressure monitor. It certainly made my blood pressure soar! I was terrified of that machine. Every minute or two it would tense its grip on my arm so tightly I was afraid it might stop my blood flowing completely. Then, just when I thought it would never stop, it released itself again. My stomach and my lower body always felt raw, like I'd been scraped out with a knife. When I looked around the recovery area there were always other bodies lying supine on their trolleys. They were so still I was afraid they might be dead. Everyone and everything looked fuzzy without my contact lenses in.

'How do you feel?' a nurse would suddenly pop her head into my line of vision, her face so close to mine I could see the fine lines tracked beneath her eyes.

'Okay,' I'd croak back, obediently, aware that my throat felt tender and dry. The green-draped nurse would summon two male porters with a quick jerk of her covered head. They would wheel me back to my room, lifting me into my bed in a sort of hammock, before taking the trolley back.

Graham would be waiting for me, a worried expression on his newly lined, sweet face, his hair jutting out in clumps where he'd been jerking his fingers through it, while walking the floor. He'd not been allowed into the operating theatre and so had gone to his parents' house, after "depositing" as the nurse called it, his semen, as if he'd ejaculated through a letterbox, then watched as his stock rose at his own private sperm bank.

Often, I'd be delayed in theatre and Graham would pace about anxiously, not knowing what was going on. My throat would always be inflamed when I came back so I could hardly gasp back whispers to his questions. I'd always be parched and desperate for a cup of tea. Then they'd bring me some food, usually a sandwich and some cake. After that a nurse would visit bringing me, in a white paper bag, all I needed for my follow-up injection: the needle; the syringe; the drug ampoule. This was to be given two days later by my doctor. The nurse would inform us how many eggs they'd recovered, telling us, 'Please phone tomorrow after ten to find out how many have fertilised. You can go home at five-thirty, as long as you've had something to eat and drink and have been to the toilet.' Then she'd rustle off.

Every time I tried to get up to use the toilet, the pain in my stomach felt like a sharp, glittering knife twisting in my guts. Even worse than that was the reek of the anaesthetic gas in my nose, throat and lungs. I always felt great green waves of sickness swell over me. Every slight movement I made caused the room to rotate around me.

I always found it difficult to get out of my hospital bed. I'd struggle up but felt so queasy and dizzy that I'd have to lie back down again to make the undulations of nausea recede, moving from overpoweringly swamping tidal waves to gently lapping ripples. I'd know I was going to vomit. My temperature would rush up the scale and I'd feel boiling, like a rumbling about-to-blow volcano. I knew if I moved, I'd be sick. That first time I vomited into the wastepaper basket! Throwing up eased the nausea but it brought back the smell and taste of the stench of the anaesthetic gas that lurked, reeking darkly in my nostrils and mouth. Then I was able to inch with trembling steps to the bathroom and use the toilet, though it stung. I'd then be able to dress myself in slow motion, my clothes, like my limbs, feeling as if they were made of granite. This caused billows of nausea to again ripple over me. I'd feel like a tiny dinghy buffeted about on a very stormy sea. I'd sit by an open window trying to gulp in air to make me feel better.

Every single time I wondered how I'd get home. It seemed ridiculously impossible, like climbing a snow-packed Ben Nevis in just my nightdress and bare feet; yet I longed for my own bed. I wanted a magical transporter out of science fiction, to beam me instantly from the hospital to my home, with no effort required on my part.

The nurses were always lovely though. They'd come to check how I was and fuss over me, bringing me a small white tablet to swallow, to stop the nausea, lilting, in a singsong voice that it was, 'No problem AT ARLLL,' if I wanted to stay the night. But I knew we'd have to pay another great wad of money we didn't have to stay in this private hospital, so made a monumental effort to reach our car, hanging onto a grey cardboard container to use as a sick bucket. I knew I was walking like a jerky puppet with a child of two pulling the strings but didn't care.

Once we were home, I'd collapse on the marshmallow-soft best bed in the whole world. Bliss!

The morning after an egg recovery was always tough. I'd wake with my stomach contracting like it had been kicked by a wild-eyed, frothing-at-the-mouth, panicking stallion. My throat would feel rubbed raw. I always had sores in my mouth. My shoulders would feel knotted with pain from the general anaesthetic trapped in my muscles. My vagina would be sore and sensitively tender, stinging when I went to the toilet.

Worse than the physical discomfort was the anxiety: how many of our eggs would fertilise into viable embryos? Next day we'd phone terrified for the result.

The day after was the embryo replacement. We'd walk from our hospital room to the operating theatre together, me in my pink slippers and white towelling dressing gown over my green hospital gown. Graham and I had to put blue hair nets over our heads, which looked and felt like J-cloths and pale blue plastic covers over our slippers and shoes, to eliminate any germs before we were allowed into the little room off the main operating theatre to view our embryos before they were replaced. I'd always approach the microscope with my heart palpitating madly, stooping to press my eyes against the cold metal viewers, terrified to touch anything in case it damaged my precious babies-to-be. The embryos always looked like bubbles joined together, like frog spawn. Sometimes they had four cells, sometimes six or, best of all, eight.

Then came the painful, embarrassing part: I had to climb up and lie on a specially designed operating table. I'd wriggle my buttocks into a particular groove, then the nurse and doctor would take the end of the table away, so that my bare bottom would be practically hanging out and my legs pressed up against two bars to keep them out of the way, giving easier access to my womb. Then the doctor would put the cold speculum into my vagina while Graham held my hand. After much twisting and fiddling about with the metal instrument and a lot of discomfort for me, he'd release the two embryos into my lonely, empty womb, shooting them in through a tiny tube.

Graham and I would always clasp hands and smile at each other at this *the* moment of conception. I'd be sure it was all over and feel so happy and relieved, despite being nakedly exposed to my very core. Then I'd be covered up and hoisted by two male porters onto a trolley, wheeled back to my room and lifted back into my bed which had now been specially adjusted so that my legs would lie higher than my head. After that I had to lie for *four* long hours, hardly moving at all before I was allowed home. I'd be given food and finally allowed to leave, feeling dizzy.

Two days later I'd go to my doctors for the "final" injection, consisting of hCG, the hormone my body would manufacture if I were pregnant. Its production would stop my body from attacking the two embryos as foreign bodies, trick it into thinking they were part of itself and so help them implant into the lining of my womb.

Then, the very worst part of all: the waiting. We felt so powerless our emotions fluctuated up and down, continually. It was *agonising*. One minute we felt certain I was pregnant; and the next, convinced I wasn't. It was a manic-depressive cycle of intense euphoria, followed by severe misery. Every night I suffered the torment of anxiety dreams. In one, I was dancing around naked in front of a crowd of my fully dressed acquaintances and embarrassing everyone. In another, I was back in my old infant school, completely grown-up but still a pupil in the class amongst dozens of five-year-old children. In yet another I was in my classroom teaching but being totally ignored by my class. Then I was taking assembly in front of a crowded school hall but when I opened my mouth not one word would emerge. I was always so glad to wake up!

Two weeks after the egg recovery was the day I was most likely to bleed. This was torture, when I kept checking for blood every ten minutes or so, like a child searching the empty railway track for an expected train. This was when I felt almost *insane* with anxiety. My moods were so volatile, I felt like I was stuck in a lift with a maniac who couldn't keep her fingers off the buttons.

'I always feel like my head is about to crack open under this pressure,' I'd complain to Graham.

He felt it too. 'It's like water torture,' he'd agree. 'That relentless drip drip drip…'

Then I'd become convinced I really *was* pregnant.

It was always at the worst time, such as when I was due back at work, that I found the blood. Then my whole world would quake on its axis, my knees shuddering, my whole-body tremoring and head reeling. The timing was always terrible. I was invariably alone; Graham having gone off to work leaving me to cope with this disaster all on my own. I would find the blood and then go off to do my job as if nothing catastrophic had happened. I'd be so convinced, would have wagered good money on it: hundreds of pounds washed away in seas of blood. I felt like God, fate, destiny had booted me in the guts. A visceral pain would seep through my being like the menstrual blood itself, spreading like a stain, tainting me and my life. I would later have to tell Graham and see the disappointment in his eyes.

I'd always want to cry but forced myself not to. I didn't want to turn up for school with bloodshot, tear-stained eyes. After all, if I couldn't have a child and it seemed more and more likely I never would, at least I had my career. Besides, I needed the money to pay for my next lot of fertility treatment. It would have been better for me if I'd been in a school with relative strangers, but I'd been there for *years:* everyone knew me. How I longed for the privacy of anonymity. Every time it failed, I had the ordeal of everyone asking me how it had gone all day long and I had to repeat the bad news over and over again, even before my beloved Graham knew, making me feel guilty to add to my misery. I used to watch their uncomprehending faces trying to be sympathetic and hear them mouth such platitudes as, 'Better luck next time!' All anybody else talked about were the fabulous family holidays they'd just been on, how marvellous their children were, and how well they'd done in their exams. I always longed to shout at them to shut up and knock their boastful heads together, but instead I had to pretend to be cheerful, as if I were not absolutely *destroyed* and that my world had not collapsed around my lifeless ears.

Each time the treatment failed I thought, *this is the worst day of my life*. I never got used to it, so it never got easier. Each time I fell into the depths of the abyss. I longed to get home but dreaded it, too. I'd have to tell Graham making him as miserable as I was but at least at home I could cry in peace, away from all these laughing people with their perfect tans and their glossy holiday photos of their cherished rosy-cheeked children.

I'd leave work as early as possible, at four, and every single time I passed my headteacher's office, strategically placed at the only exit, she'd spot me and say something like, 'Put your feet up!' I'm sure she intended it to be reassuring but it made me feel insane with anger.

Another of my colleagues would ask, 'Are you going out tonight?' a snide comment on my unusually early departure. I'd just have emerged hurriedly from the toilet where I'd have witnessed close-up the ghastly obvious signs of miscarriage: not just fresh raspberry-red blood but black lumps and clots, sticky, like the skin of *dead babies.* Was I going out? As if I had anything to celebrate! So, I'd just fix them with my cold, tormented eyes and twist my hurt mouth into a terse, 'No.'

As soon as I drove out of the car park I'd start crying. I'd have been holding my pain deep inside me all day and now it would erupt. I really should have pulled the car over for safety reasons, as I couldn't see well enough to drive. But I never did. I dared not stop. I was afraid if I did, I'd never start driving again, never move from that spot.

When Graham came home, I'd cry all over him. I felt emotionally crazed, wailing that it was never going to work, we'd never have a baby and Graham would agree. We felt like we'd been cursed. I felt like a failure as a woman. All human beings must do is reproduce themselves and I couldn't even do that. I understood people who drank themselves to death or took drugs: all their hope was gone. I tried to think about people worse off than myself, those who had cancer, who knew they were dying but I couldn't because I envied them: death seemed a blessed relief from the devastating emotional pain I felt. How could I go on? Without a child there was no life, no hope, no future. What was the point? My body longed for a child with a palpable physical ache and my womb, my heart and my arms felt empty.

Graham had the typically masculine response every time the treatment failed: he blamed other people and wanted to lash out at them. My typically feminine response was to blame *myself,* turning my anger inwards.

Yet, after it failed and I'd cried hysterically, I always slept better than I had for months: the release of all that tension and emotion.

I had to wait for two normal menstruations to give my body the chance to get back to normal after all the fertility drugs. Then our lives once again became a frenzied blur of hospital visits, injections, trips to the doctor and blood tests, like a film watched on fast forward.

Finally, after *eight* long years of trying to have a baby and intensive fertility procedures, we knew we only had three frozen embryos left. We didn't know if we could stand to have any more treatment. Our emotions were on a continuous rise and fall cycle. I always found the blood in my knickers when I was alone or at work where I couldn't talk about it, and that in itself felt like a cruel curse. I tried to keep the tragic news to myself, but everyone could see from my distraught face what had happened. I thought (and I may be wrong, but this *was* how I felt) that some people did seem to want to see me break down and cry, but I vowed that I wouldn't. My private misery was not going to be paraded for the public entertainment of people who had what I so desperately wanted: a baby. Child-rich parents could never, ever understand.

I plodded on with my life, trying not to think or feel. I was a dead woman walking around. I didn't want to be myself anymore or live my own life. At school I could play the role of being the efficient, caring teacher and I lost myself in that. My career progressed and it partly pleased me, but it also upset me: why was I killing myself for other peoples' children when the stress of the job was probably what was preventing me from conceiving my own? Without a child my life was empty. Nothing made up for it. Always deep inside there was a child-shaped hole that only a baby could fill.

When we arrived for our embryo replacement, one of the nurses ushered us into an interview room. This was unusual. Our inner alarm bells started ringing loudly and we exchanged anxious glances. The unfamiliar nurse didn't look into our eyes but at our mouths as she glanced from one of us to the other, mumbling awkwardly, 'I'm sorry to have to tell you but one of your embryos…' she paused, as if to remember the appropriate quote from the handbook, 'has not survived the freeze-thaw process.'

My face must have reacted instantly for Graham stared at me, horrified. 'You mean it's *dead,*' I said, flatly. I felt a sudden overpowering urge to cry, feeling my eyes prickling with tears.

'You still have *two* lovely, healthy embryos left and we can replace them today,' the nurse reminded us, in a stridently cheerful voice. Despite the tiny glimmer of hope, we remained shocked and saddened. I was reeling. This truly would be the final time that we would ever come to this hospital with hope in our hearts. It certainly was my very *last* chance.

Later, in the viewing room, I stared at my final two embryos through the microscope. This reassured me during the pain and embarrassment of having them replaced inside me. My recalcitrant womb was twisted back this time, so Doctor Briscoe had to clamp the neck of it to hold it in position. It was excruciatingly painful. This thing that felt like a metal trap for catching rabbits snapped onto it and then gripped my womb so tightly that I felt I might blackout from the pain. But I was strong. At last, the embryos were shot into my womb.

I felt ashamed to be the only naked person in the room, under my loose, green hospital gown. I hated the dazzling white lights concentrated on what were once my most secret, intimate parts. It was horrible and uncomfortable. 'This will *never, ever* replace sex as a sensible person's choice of how to conceive a baby,' I told Graham later, grimly. It really was nothing like conception should be, that magically mystical, private moment of joy, pleasure and bonding between two people deeply in love. Instead, it was sterile, painful and degrading, thanks to the insertion of a metal instrument under a spotlight with witnesses. I felt such a failure which was why, it seemed, the doctors and nurses were always poking around inside me, as if searching for that elusive baby who was never, ever there.

At last the ordeal was over and I was manhandled onto a trolley and wheeled back to my room, a strange trip of white ceilings and blazing lights. I remember the undersides of people's faces and being pushed and jiggled into lifts, along endless corridors past staring eyes. I felt dizzy and spinning with disorientation. Then I had to wriggle off the trolley and on to the bed, wondering if my longed-for baby would ever come.

I suddenly realised that other women didn't talk to me about their own children anymore, in fact, the only ones brave enough to mention children to me at all were those who could not conceive. It was as if I'd joined a secret club "Women Who Could NOT Have Babies" but, just like Groucho Marx, I didn't want to be a member of this club, the only one that would have me: I wanted to be a member of "Happy Mother's Club", but nature kept slamming the door on my eager face.

Yet, once again, like an old lady who hears a familiar tune and is deluged with memories, I was *sure* that I really was pregnant this time. In fact, never had I felt more confident. It felt so real this time and different somehow. It was my third cycle of IVF: could it really be third and final time lucky?

Chapter 12

A very bad joke

On the Saturday morning I woke at six. Immediately I thrust my hand between my legs: NO BLOOD! We had never actually reached our contact day without bleeding before. I had that feeling I used to have as a five-year-old, waking up on Christmas morning, that something wonderful and exciting was about to happen. I hardly dared move or breathe. I knew as soon as I tried to get up that Graham, a very light sleeper, would wake up too and urge me to do a pregnancy test. So instead, I lay in bed, too thrilled yet frightened to do anything.

Finally, when I couldn't stand it one single second longer, I edged out of bed as quietly as possible, inch by creaking inch and scurried to the bathroom. Immediately I checked for blood: nothing. I needed a container to hold my urine, so I raced downstairs and grabbed the empty cottage cheese carton I kept the biros in, by the phone. This would do. I tipped out the pens and clutching it to my heart, ran back upstairs as quietly as I could. I sat on the toilet, the receptacle clamped between my thighs and let my urine burst out of me, collecting it carefully. I dunked the pen-shaped pregnancy indicator in. I didn't need to check the instructions: I'd done countless pregnancy tests. If I was pregnant, both windows would develop thin, blue lines.

I gazed breathlessly, kneeling on the hard pale wood of the bathroom floor. I felt my heart pounding powerfully. Slowly, minutely, I watched, millimetre by millimetre as my urine rose up the test, sluggishly, the first "control" window developed a thin, blue line then, indolently creeping, before my astonished, urging eyes, the other window developed a definite blue line too. I blinked. My eyes grew so fuzzy and blurred, I could hardly see let alone breathe. I blinked again. Yes, there it was: I was PREGNANT! I remained crouching, stunned and disbelieving. The next second, I found myself dashing back into my bedroom, brandishing the test aloft, like a magic wand emitting sparks. Graham was already sitting up in bed, round-eyed, hardly daring to look.

'I'M PREGNANT!' I shouted, as if he was in an adjoining room, not right next to me.

'LOOK!' I held the test under his stunned brown eyes, not quite steadily. He grabbed it to hold it still and gaped at it himself, eyes popping. I threw my arms around his neck and we kissed quickly, distractedly, in amazement and delight. We couldn't believe the proof of our own eyes and kept staring at the test afraid it would change or disappear.

'Aren't there two tests in the packet?' gasped Graham. (He knew there were, as I had fruitlessly done enough of the things and bulk bought them, despite their high cost.) 'Let me watch it change with my own eyes,' he pleaded. My skin thrilled all over, in anticipation of the joy of watching our very first affirmative pregnancy test turn positive together. I entrusted the precious first one to him like it was the crown jewels and ran to the bathroom, wrestled the second one out of the blue-and-white box and the silver-foil wrapping and brought it, with the carton of my urine, into the bedroom. I let Graham dip the second test in, which he did, very carefully. We both gawped, saucer-eyed and enraptured as yet again, *both* windows developed blue lines. We goggled at each other, open-mouthed. *Two* positive pregnancy tests: the first two we had ever had in our whole lives! I felt as if I shone with happiness, all warm and glowing inside, like I'd swallowed sunshine. I swept the pink curtains back and gazed out of the bedroom window at our lush, green back garden and said to Graham, 'This is the most beautiful day I've ever seen!' I smiled out at my garden, and it seemed to sparkle back at me in its rich, succulent fertility: *I* was like that now. Before I'd been a barren desert but now, I was throbbing with new life.

We spent the next three hours marvelling at our astonishing luck, not knowing what to do, waiting impatiently for the time to pass quickly, and then, at nine-thirty, we set off for the hospital for our official pregnancy test there.

Graham and I expected a blare of trumpets and the thunder of drums as we walked in, but everything was just as normal. Mary, one of the nurses we knew well, after our three cycles of IVF at this hospital, was on duty. I rather breathlessly unwrapped the two positive pregnancy tests from their protective white tissue, with quite a flourish, to show her. I expected gulps of wonderment, tears of rapture, screams and hugs but she just commented in her measured, nurse-like way, 'Commercial pregnancy tests are usually fairly accurate,' as if it was every day that I discovered I was pregnant. She took the blood from a vein in my left arm. 'I'll phone you with the results as soon as I can, about eleven-thirty,' she promised.

We didn't know what to do with ourselves while we waited.

'We could do the weekly shop,' suggested Graham, practical as ever. So off we went to Asda and stocked up on food, smiling compulsively at each other as we wended around the aisles, nursing our secret joy to ourselves.

We waited in agony. 'It is good news,' said Mary, when she finally rang. 'The test result *is* positive, so many congratulations. Lorna needs to come in for a scan in three weeks to confirm the foetal heartbeat. We'll send you a date and time.' Graham put the phone down and we jumped up and down hugging, like three-year-olds, ecstatic to have our own results confirmed by the hospital's blood test.

'You are definitely clinically, medically, officially PREGNANT!' Graham bellowed in a crescendo at me. I blinked back: it was so hard to believe, after all these eight desperate years. I felt my heart full-to-bursting with exultation, feeling nothing could ever hurt or harm me again. We were going to have a child. I knew I would never be unhappy again.

But as usual, I was being far too extreme. Once the rapture faded, I again felt awful. I was still waiting to bleed, as in the bad old days of the fertility treatment. Every time I went to the toilet (and I seemed to go more than ever now I was pregnant) I checked for blood and my heart was jittery. I was also finding it hard to sleep because of my alternate bouts of excitement and anxiety. Every so often I did feel that strong rush of euphoria, when everything in my world seemed to look better and be illuminated, as if an intense golden light was being shined upon it and I couldn't believe how happy I was; but I soon plunged back to the ground with a thump. Every twinge in my stomach I thought was the beginning of a miscarriage. I knew, grimly, that the next eight months were going to be very long and full of anxiety. I had so longed to be an expectant mother and now I was I hated it! I felt that nature had played a very bad joke on me.

When I was six weeks pregnant, I was shopping in town, feeling a happy, fruitful part of the whole resonating throng of people. Then I nipped into John Lewis to use their toilet and found blood in my knickers, exactly the sort that I always had when I was about to start my period. To compound my misery, I also had stomach cramps that felt like menstrual pains, complete with vibrating womb! I forced myself home to rest, pretending that everything was fine, even though my heart was breaking up with fear. I didn't even tell Graham because I really had nothing to tell him: I'd had no more bleeding. I went to bed immediately and waited, stiff with stark desolation.

When I woke up after a nightmare-packed sleep, I expected to find my knickers, which I'd cautiously left on, soaked with blood but there was none. I had to tell Graham as he'd noticed how depressed I seemed. He called a doctor to come out on his rounds while I stayed in bed. Black-suited Doctor Webster arrived, after a two hour wait and felt my stomach.

'Your womb is not in spasm,' he informed me, reassuringly. 'You'll probably be fine. Stay in bed and don't go back to work for a week.'

I felt incredibly relieved at his pronouncements. I felt even more reassured that the two pregnancy tests I'd sent Graham to the chemist for first thing that morning, were both still positive. I kept comforting myself with the mantra, 'The baby is fine, so far, so good.' I was also extremely grateful to be told to stay off work for a week as I'd been feeling totally exhausted.

That week I was off work my eating habits went berserk. I couldn't stand even the smell of food I normally enjoyed eating. I would suddenly lust after something I usually loathed, like a Cornish pasty. I would wrest one from a pack in the freezer (always plenty there as Graham loved them) and heat it up in the microwave, pressing my nose against the vibrating glass, urging it, 'Faster!' Then I'd cram it into my salivating mouth, still so radiation-frazzled hot that it burnt my tongue, gobbling it down, desperately. Then I felt terribly ill. I alternated constantly between these extremes of feeling sick or ravenous with strange cravings. There seemed to be no in-between stages at all. It was very odd, like an alien life-form had hijacked my body.

The term "morning sickness" really annoyed me. It sounded so negligible, as if someone got up in the morning, felt a bit nauseous for a few dizzy seconds, shrugged it off and then got on with their full and busy life. I tried to explain it to Graham, to his mother and sister, to my mum, and all who claimed never to have experienced such a thing. 'It's like being seasick,' I told them, 'On a ship you can never get off.' I felt terrible all the time, as if I could vomit at any moment. I felt frightened to do anything or go anywhere in case I was sick (not that I felt like going anywhere or doing anything. I felt far too ill for that).

The fear of throwing up was disabling. The shame of losing control of my body in public was more than I could bear. I stayed in as much as I could, forced to abandon my teaching job. Home was the only place I felt safe, where I had my sick bucket and my toilet always available for emergencies.

Every time I vomited was the same. I'd lie, unmoving, while sickness flooded me in waves, rising and falling like a boiling, choppy sea. I'd lie very still, knowing that as soon as I moved, the green nausea would be unleashed. Then, when I couldn't stand it an instant longer, I moved and it all erupted in projectile *spurts*. I was racked again and again, emptied out, choking, eyes watering, blisteringly hot and then, suddenly cold.

I'd lie on the floor, cooling my hot cheek against the porcelain base of the toilet. What a strange shape my toilet pedestal was, I thought. I'd never had this ant's view before. The rumble and rush, the gurgle and roar of the flushing toilet was so violent. I shook all over. The pipe hummed; the water glugged and burbled, like my acid stomach.

I could only tell Graham the truth: I'd never felt worse in my entire life. It wasn't just the constant nausea, the feeling I was about to be sick: the actual vomiting itself was vile. It was frightening, not like normal throwing up. It didn't seem to stop, feeding on itself, cannibalistically. It made my eyes water and my hands shake. I gulped in air, desperately. When I'd finally paused, my stomach vibrated, sore and over-exerted, stretched to breaking point. I felt weak and worried about the baby. How could the poor child possibly be all right and getting enough nutrients when I vomited up everything I ate or drank? But it was such a relief to get rid of it all, to wipe out that burning nausea collecting in my throat and that windy bloating in my stomach. The hot, scary knowledge that if I just turned my head or bent down for something, I would be sick, kept me fixed bolt upright in my chair. I was traumatised by the hot sweatiness of it, the embarrassment, the feeling of doom that it would go on forever until the end of my life.

And then there was the awful leaden tiredness I felt. I'd thought I'd felt weary before but I'd never experienced exhaustion like this. My mind and body felt numb with it, as it just fell upon me like a dead weight every so often. Suddenly I could do nothing. I had so little energy I couldn't even think properly. I felt sickened. It took all the strength and willpower I possessed to crawl up the stairs, clean my ghastly white face and brush my yellowing teeth.

When I crashed gratefully into bed, always in the very early evenings around eight, I'd sigh with deliverance. I longed to sleep but felt somehow beyond it, as if I was already too drained for it. Blackbirds were still piping outside and children playing riotously in the beer garden of The Red Lion. Graham would be hosing the flowers or cutting the grass or inside, watching football on the blaring television. It seemed so unnatural to be lying in bed, consumed with fatigue, yet not able to sleep. Everyone else's life was going on as normal but mine had completely stopped. All I seemed to do was dither about the house and feel ill and exhausted.

In bed I felt roasted and uncomfortable. I couldn't lie on my back as I felt sick or on my side as I crushed my arm. Eventually I'd doze off but then I'd wake up again, an hour later, desperate for the toilet. I'd dash to the bathroom. Then I'd feel dizzily sick and must rush back to lie down, to quell the nausea threatening to engulf me. I had perfected the unusual but necessary technique of using the toilet while I had my head down in the wash basin next to it, both orifices spewing forth in a great gush together, like a disgusting duet. I didn't even dare to think about the baby being harmed by all this. And so, it went on, day after relentless night. Also, I'd developed two gum infections, one on my left lower jaw and one on my upper right, so even if I'd been able to eat normally, I couldn't because it hurt too much.

To add to my torment I looked awful. My breasts seemed swollen to many times their normal size. I lugged them around, like enormous virulently pink weapons that no bra or top could contain. They kept trying to escape out of wherever they were buried, like two burrowing moles. My stomach was an elephantine mound, protruding out of my clothes, entering any room well before I did. My hair was abominable. I'd read in a pregnancy magazine (the usual off-putting beautiful mother-to-be on the cover) that hair dye or bleach could penetrate through a woman's skin, get into her bloodstream and harm the developing baby, so I'd not had my hair done at all since I became pregnant. I sported one solid inch of dark roots with straw-like bleached ends. I looked so appalling I was afraid to glance into a mirror and be horrified by my own death-mask white skin and wanted it to be covered in black material, like the Victorians did when in mourning.

I was supposed to feel better once I'd passed the twelve-week mark, everyone said but I did not. My vomiting just continued. All I could do was complain, then I felt ashamed of myself for moaning, but I just couldn't help it: I felt terrible. I had to keep reminding myself that I was really delighted to be pregnant; after all, it had taken me eight years and thousands of pounds to get into this *hellish* state.

I was still having "morning sickness" (and afternoon, evening and night sickness, too) at sixteen weeks. Graham asked me, at four-thirty one morning as I was vomiting for the fifth time, 'Can I get you anything?'

'Yes. Get me a doctor,' I told him, weakly, between heaving spews. I felt so dreadful I thought it couldn't possibly just be morning sickness: it *must* be stomach cancer! No wonder poor Charlotte Brontë died of it. My whole body ached: I had a ravaged stomach and a raw throat. My ribs hurt from the continuous inside pressure on them: I even thought I may have cracked one or two from hanging over the side of my bed to vomit so violently. The next day I always felt so fragile and sensitive. Even the merest whiff of a scent of certain foods could set me off again. I couldn't go anywhere in my black Fiesta as the smell of the interior and the motion of it made me be sick after a few minutes.

I dragged myself to see the midwife at my doctor's surgery on the high street. I lumbered into her room, ashen-faced. 'I'm seventeen weeks,' I told her, desperately. 'Surely this sickness will stop soon. All my friends and family say it should have stopped at twelve weeks.'

The midwife's tired features took on a pitying look. 'Oh no,' she said. 'I've known plenty of women to go through their whole pregnancy vomiting.'

I dragged myself home to *die*.

Then, suddenly, when I was eighteen weeks, the sickness eased off. 'At last,' I told Graham, delightedly, 'Now I can really begin to enjoy my pregnancy.'

As soon as I heard the stranger's voice on the phone, *I knew*. It was the call I'd been dreading since I'd had the "triple test" on my blood. I realised the medical staff wouldn't contact me unless I was in deep trouble.

'It's the hospital here,' said the unfamiliar voice. My heart suddenly plunged to the back of my heels, like a lift would plummet if the cables were slashed. 'Your triple test has come back and I'm afraid you are high risk. There's a one-in-forty chance there's maybe something wrong. The investigation showed an elevated probability of spina bifida and Down's syndrome. Why don't you come in for counselling? Are you free this afternoon?'

I couldn't think clearly, I felt so shocked. I knew Graham was in work, probably busy in a meeting. I supposed he could take leave for the next morning, as it was an emergency, so I said we'd both come in for advice then. I'd managed to keep calm whilst on the phone but the instant the nurse rang off, I collapsed on the floor, violently sobbing. I rang Graham right away but as soon as I heard his voice, I suddenly couldn't manage to speak coherently. He panicked completely on the other end of the phone, thinking I was miscarrying as I spoke and reassured me, 'I'm coming home right now. I'll be there within the hour.'

I paced around the house until he came, dragging my shattered heart around in my leaden feet. I knew I'd feel better with Graham there. I didn't know what to think. Surely the hospital wouldn't bother pregnant women with awful prognostications unless they were sure there was something badly wrong with the baby? I couldn't believe it. Not us. Not after *all* we'd been through. How could this be happening? Surely life couldn't be so cruel.

Graham arrived looking bloodless and breathless, having run all the way home uphill from the train station. He couldn't believe our bad luck either. He drove me to the hospital at face-distorting speed, after I rang them back to say we were coming in straight away, after all.

Graham and I sat in the crowded waiting room like two strangers in a lift, not even daring to make eye contact or speak. All around us babies and toddlers played and laughed, and pregnant women came and went, smiling smugly to themselves. The nursing sister who was also a trained counsellor came to fetch us, ushering us into a private room. We talked for a whole hour. She described to us many cases where the triple test had not been right.

'They are only seventy-per-cent accurate, I'm afraid,' she informed us, her bright blue eyes glistening with sympathy. 'Why don't I book you in for an amniocentesis test which could tell you for sure if something is wrong or not? In the amnio, the doctor puts a very fine needle into your womb, to draw off some amniotic fluid containing a few of the baby's cells...'

'Isn't that dangerous?' I asked, horrified.

'The procedure has a one-in-fifteen chance of causing a miscarriage. Then the baby's cells are cultured in the lab, and you have to wait three weeks before you can count the chromosomes, but it will give you a definite result.'

We talked on and on. Eventually the counsellor said she'd "pencil us in" for an amniocentesis on the Wednesday, after our rather delayed eighteen-week scan. Then, if we decided we didn't want it, we could phone to cancel.

Graham and I went home and debated it endlessly. I felt so depressed. Really, I was having the pregnancy from *hell*, and I was only five months in! I felt I had a black, satanic cloud suspended over me. I might miscarry after the amniocentesis or I might be diagnosed as carrying a disabled child and then, what would we do? We'd be offered, the counsellor said, a 'medical termination of pregnancy,' or in other words, an abortion. How could we do that? And how could I ever get pregnant again? And, even if I miraculously could, who was to say the same thing wouldn't happen once more; or even worse?

Somehow, I managed to sleep the night before, worn out with worries. But I jolted awake with a jump. What had awakened me? Everything seemed quiet. I listened, my heart vibrating fast. Graham slept on heavily beside me. I stretched out a tentative, trembling hand to flick on the bedside light and look at my watch: 3.05 a.m. Why was it always three a.m. when I awoke in turmoil and sweating with worries? My fears, restrained in sunlit hours, had now grown to dizzying dimensions and expanded to fill my whole gruesome universe: my baby fears; painful disease; dying; death, all stalked the labyrinths of my mind and were multiplying with dazzling speed, like cancer cells. I stared in misery at my bedroom wall while Graham slept, racked with anxiety about what this day might bring.

Chapter 13

Incredibly unbelievable

The next day I was up early to follow the hospital's instructions closely. I drank the one-and-a-half pints of water one hour before so that I'd be perfectly ready for my scan and amniocentesis. If anything went wrong, I vowed, it wouldn't be because of me. I was ready and prepared, wearing my favourite maternity dress, the black one with the plum and lilac-coloured flowers on it, for courage and luck.

Tiger, next door's cat, was waiting on my doorstep that morning, as she always was when I found myself in emotional turmoil. I let her in, as usual, and she bounded in but instead of rushing to rub herself all over my ankles, as she routinely did, she ran away from me, right around the wooden coffee table and back out of the front door. This was very bizarre; but I had other worries.

I sat in the waiting room with Graham, apprehensive and preoccupied. I was glad to be called in by the sonographer, wanting to get it over with. I had to take my dress off and put a green hospital gown on over my bra and knickers. I lay on the scanning table and the sonographer squeezed cold gel on to my stomach and started the machine humming. The scanner skimmed lightly over my greasy bump. The lights were off in the room so the sonographer could see the pictures on the monitor more clearly and the darkness gave a strange feeling of intimate closeness. I watched the glow from the screen flicker on her sad, drawn face, her black bobbed hair, her almond-shaped green darting eyes, her tightly compressed mouth.

'Is everything all right?' I blurted out, involuntarily.

'You'll have to forgive me. I've got a lot of measuring to do, so I really can't chat.'

She didn't look into my eyes but over my right shoulder. I felt a creeping unease. Surely the woman should have said immediately that everything was fine, like the two previous sonographers at my six- and twelve-week scans. I tried to calm myself. After all, I had never had an eighteen-week scan before; never at this hospital; never with this sonographer. Maybe this was normal, and I was foolish to feel this mounting alarm.

'I'm sorry. It's just that I'm very anxious.' Sounds just seemed to erupt out of my mouth, as if I had no control over them.

The sonographer continued gazing at the monitor and I carried on staring at the woman's face, strangely illuminated by the radiating screen, searching for clues, even answers; but the sonographer's face remained a sphinx-like mask. Surely everything was fine, I thought, desperately. If (I hardly dared think it) something looked badly wrong with the baby, as I had feared last night in my worst nightmare scenario, the sonographer would not still be concentrating on the screen and measuring?

'Is your husband with you?' said the woman, in a perfectly neutral voice.

'Yes. He's in the waiting room.'

'What is his name?'

'Graham.'

'I'll just go and get him.'' She slid away as if she was on roller skates.

Oh no, I thought. Why hadn't the sonographer shown me the baby on the screen? Why hadn't she reassured me? Why had she very deliberately turned the monitor off before she left? She was several prolonged minutes collecting Graham. She was probably telling him some bad news outside so he can comfort me, I thought.

But when, at last, Graham came in, he smiled buoyantly at me, a normal, encouraging grin. For an instant I took courage from this.

But then I heard the sonographer's voice, as if it was coming from far away. 'I've got some bad news for you. I can't find a heartbeat.'

'*So... my baby is dead,*' I said. The words fell so heavily from my mouth into the silence of the room I thought they would surely smash right through the concrete floor. The bells of warning that had been tinkling far down in the depths of my head were now tolling loudly enough to make my ears bleed. Yet although everything, including my heart seemed to have stopped dead, it was a strange relief to hear the words I'd most feared spoken out loud. Somehow it seemed both incredibly unbelievable, yet also inevitable, like I'd known all along that this was going to happen. It was exactly how I had been throughout my whole pregnancy. On the one hand, I had been very positive, thinking everything would go smoothly: but, at the same time, every stomach twinge I had I'd thought was a miscarriage; every time I went to the toilet, I checked, terrified, for blood. Even when announcing to people the wonderful news that I was pregnant, a little warning voice in my head kept asking, "How long will it last?"

Now I knew, only *five months.*

A weird, gasping noise came from Graham. I moved my head to look at him, feeling like I was moving in slow-motion. I was puzzled to see tears spilling down Graham's face. He had to take his gold-rimmed glasses off, as he was blinded, to wipe his eyes with the back of his hand, like a five-year-old boy. I desperately wanted to say, "I'm *so sorry* Graham," but no sound would come out of my shocked mouth.

'All our hopes and dreams,' gulped Graham, pitifully, between sobs. I stretched out my left hand, very slowly, amazed I could still move it, and placed it on the side of his wet, dear face, tenderly, while he wept. A nurse's hand passed him a tissue. I turned my head slowly, painfully, to stare at her, bewildered. When had *she* come into the room? I felt cold, as if transported miles away, distanced from it all, like it was happening to someone else, knowing instinctively that I had to keep strong for the horror that was to come.

Both the nurse and the sonographer were making animal, comforting noises in their throats. 'You're very stoic,' the nurse told me, with an approving nod.

I leadenly rotated my frozen face towards her. 'I think I'm in shock,' I muttered. I gazed at Graham, tears leaking in a deluge down his white cheeks. The thought came into my head that I had known him for ten whole years, and I had never, *ever* seen him cry before. There was something unbearable about this strapping man who never cried sobbing uncontrollably in front of us three tearless women.

We were shepherded to a special room, set aside for counselling. The doctor who was scheduled to perform the amniocentesis talked to us for a long time, as did the nurse. I watched their mouths open and close and heard sounds of people talking but nothing was getting through to me. I felt like one of those high-security burglar systems where the alarm had been triggered and immediately my metal shutters came clanging down.

After what could have been moments or hours, we were taken to the "compassionate suite." It was on the maternity floor but hidden away in the corner, far from the newly delivered mothers and babies. Yet another white-coated doctor arrived and described what was to happen. The horror of this *did* penetrate, as it was even worse than I had feared. I had naively assumed that they would put me to sleep and take the dead baby from my womb, but the doctor said I was too far advanced in pregnancy for that: they were going to induce me into labour so that I would give birth naturally to my dead baby.

I had hoped that this, at least, I would be spared: but it seemed that I was to be spared nothing.

I'm not ready for this yet, I felt like screaming but not one word would come out of my mouth. I hadn't attended any antenatal classes: I did not know one thing about labour or what to expect, not even having read that far in my pregnancy book. Anyway, I was given no options: the impression I was given was that this was how it had to be. I felt completely closed down. I was nearly comatose but still intensely aware of everything around me: every person; every word; every look; every gesture, though none of it made any sense. I desperately wanted to respond but could not.

I slowly wrote a list for Graham, and he went home to get the things I needed for my unexpected stay in hospital.

I sat on a blue chair in the compassionate suite. I could not cry, and I could not move. I stayed in that hospital room, rigid with shock, the motionless centre of a cyclone of activity suddenly raging around me. Still, I sat on, stunned. A voice kept repeating in my head, "The baby is dead! The baby is dead!" It went on relentlessly. Nevertheless, I could hardly believe it.

On his way out of the compassionate suite, poor Graham had to walk through a huge group of rowdy, delighted people holding the strings of helium-filled shiny silver balloons bobbing aloft, while carrying armfuls of gaudy magenta and cerise flowers. The garish colours made his eyes sting, he told me much later. The crowd were drinking pink champagne and eating cake. He felt himself hellishly trapped in a party on the ward to celebrate the safe birth of a longed-for child. He absorbed the sights and sounds without looking or hearing and an awful bitterness rose and choked his throat. He couldn't help thinking: why us? Why not them? They've probably already got other children. All we wanted was *one* healthy child. Was that too much to ask? We are CURSED!

He drove home to get me all I needed on my list, though miserable to his very core. He closed his eyes as he walked past the baby's room, the one we had so carefully decorated and furnished for our much-wanted child. Soon he would have to clear it out to save me from having to do it. He would hide all the baby things away, so that I would not have to see them. But not now. He knew he wasn't strong enough to do it on this dreadful day.

When Graham returned two hours later, he found me still sitting, as if turned to stone on the same blue chair on which he'd left me.

Another white-coated blur of a doctor brought a consent form for me to sign, giving my permission to be induced after intrauterine death. He told me that the baby looked, according to the scan, as if he had stopped developing between sixteen and seventeen weeks. He did not know why, but if we allowed the hospital to do tests on him once he was born, then they might be able to find out. I longed to say "I want you to find out exactly why my child died" but I still could not speak. Nobody seemed even to notice that I could not move or make one sound. They were all too busy scurrying around doing their various tasks.

The doctor took nine separate vials of my blood. I didn't think I had that much blood in my whole body. No wonder I felt completely drained and sadly empty.

'We'll give you a good M.O.T,' the nurse smiled.

I just sat there, blankly. I felt I would not, could not object, even if someone sawed off my right foot. I could not weep one tear or utter one word: I was completely frozen and numb.

Having requested my medical records from the hospital, I found out years later that when my baby died, they tested me for chlamydia. They'd already routinely tested me for syphilis while I was pregnant. They also tested me for lupus, my glucose levels for diabetes, leukaemia in a blood coagulation test, and other cancers in a tumour markers report. They even took vaginal swabs, which I don't even remember them doing, to test for vaginitis, lactobacillus and vaginal flora. All the results came back negative as the consultant Mr Ali told me, except for a recent virus I had contracted and didn't even know I had. The culprit was called Parvovirus B19 1gM antibodies. I read this in the copies of my medical records sent to my doctor's surgery, though at the time they failed to inform me that this was what killed my baby and very nearly finished me off, too, with grief.

A nurse opened the door as I sat rooted to that blue chair in the compassionate suite, and I heard a child bawl further down the corridor. *My baby will never cry,* I thought and, just for one second, I felt my face crumple but still the tears would not come. I was afraid that once I started sobbing, I might never stop.

At least the mystery of Tiger's strange behaviour that morning was explained: she must have smelt or even sensed that the baby was dead and, in her distress, had to rush away.

Another doctor came in to begin the induction into labour at two p.m. I had to lie back on the pink-flowered duvet on the double bed, while he gave me a vigorous internal examination and rubbed prostaglandin gel on the neck of my womb to soften it and make it open. He also placed a Cervagem pessary at the very back using Gemeprost to start labour. It was, even in my distant state, embarrassingly intimate and painful. My poor womb vibrated wildly for the next half hour. Graham was shocked when he felt it through my black dress but then it stopped: it did not seem to want to give up its treasure. Different doctors did this whole torturous routine right through the night every three hours until two a.m. My waters broke into the toilet in the bathroom en suite, just before five a.m. Then the contractions pulsated increasingly strongly and became more frequent. A blue-uniformed nurse gave me pethidine to ease the pain and I vomited copiously and continuously throughout that never-ending dreadful night. Then the drugs made me feel sleepy and I was so exhausted that I dozed a little. But the pain became too much to bear again, and I was given gas and air. At eight thirty I felt an overpowering compulsion to use the toilet, so went into the en suite bathroom. I was all alone as Graham was sleeping and the midwife was with someone else. I fitted the bedpan tray I'd been given over the toilet bowl as the midwife had instructed me and bore down hard into that. I felt all sorts of things slither out of me in one enormous gush.

I felt suddenly terrified to look down but knew I must force my eyes. When I did, there was my baby, a perfect little boy, thin, white, lying in a pool of brown liquid and blood. The umbilical cord protruded from his swollen stomach, thin as a strand of spaghetti. His skinny arms had fallen helplessly outwards and back, away from his body. I gawped down at my baby and he stared back at me. I gazed into his open dead eyes, the same shape and colour as mine and I knew what horror was.

I'd never seen a dead person before.

I didn't dare touch my child, afraid of how cold he might feel, how lifeless. All through that endless night of labour, I'd hoped for a miracle; that the sonographer was wrong, that my baby would be born alive. But he was indisputably dead: even I could see and accept that now.

I called out for Graham to wake him up, waddling back into the room, holding the bed-pan tray between my legs, my lost child lying in it. He yelled for assistance. Two midwives rushed in and helped me lie back on the bed.

One whisked my baby away.

I never saw him again.

The afterbirth would not come out, the other told me. She tried to yank it out with forceps but failed. I was bleeding heavily and was rushed into the operating theatre for a dilatation and curettage procedure to scrape all that was left of my baby from my womb. I had to sign a consent form for "removal of retained placenta".

A green-eyed Irish nurse hovered by me as I came round, groggy from the anaesthetic.

'And isn't your tiny baby in good company in heaven this week to be sure?' she asked me, crossing herself, devoutly. Both Princess Diana *and* Mother Theresa had died that terrible week in 1997. I had a sudden vision of my poor boy, chubby, pink and bouncingly alive now, nestled in Princess Diana's loving arms, her beautiful face radiating compassionate joy and Mother Theresa's craggy, monkey face smiling, as if both were saying, "Your baby is safe, now." But then I fell back down into my present reality. There were to be no more comforting fantasies for me.

I turned my whole body away to face the blank white wall and willed myself to die.

Yet something was keeping me going. Deep inside I had a faith that this was not really the end of my dreams for a baby. I had conceived before so the chances where I would again. I still had a tiny germ of hope inside me that things would get better.

Chapter 14

Senseless with grief

As I was taken into the operating theatre, Graham went home again. He took all the children's things out of the baby's room and couldn't help but cry as he held the tiny white cardigan that my mum had knitted for our new-born baby. My boy would have been all cosy in this, he thought, as his tears ran, ignored. He couldn't bear to think about his lost child being so cold and the fact that nothing could ever warm him up again. He folded the cardigan carefully and placed it in a black bin bag with the other clothes and toys. It didn't take him long to clear the room. Thank god we had been cautious in our preparations, he confided to me later, but the new pine wardrobe and chest of drawers and the beech rocking-chair would have to stay. We would make use of them, perhaps, at some time in the future, he told himself, should this massive, throbbing grief ever subside.

He hid the black bin bag containing all the baby clothes and toys in the spare room where I wouldn't come across it. Relieved that his sad duty was complete, he went back to the hospital, to wait for me.

I was brought back to him by lunchtime. I didn't feel sick after the anaesthetic, probably because I'd vomited up every scrap I'd eaten beforehand during my nightmarish hours of labour. My throat felt redly raw, probably from the breathing tube put down it. I could only whisper in a gravelly voice, not that I had anything to express. There was nothing to say. It was painful for me to sit down; I was bleeding so heavily. By three p.m. I wanted to go home, feeling there was no reason to stay. They had been kind to us in the hospital but now I felt exhausted and wanted to get home, hoping I would sleep forever and never have to wake up. I couldn't relax in there with people in and out all the time. I got dressed and packed my blue case and finally, after some toast and tea, one of the doctors gave us permission to go. I sent Graham to the shop to buy a box of Quality Street to thank the staff on the ward, and then we were allowed to leave.

Graham and I were so relieved to get home. I felt that only there could I unwind and crumble when I'd had to be so calm and strong in the hospital, to get through my ordeal. We sat in the baby's room, Graham on the brown beech rocking-chair and me in my grandmother's armchair. Finally, I could *cry*, a choking flood of tears.

Graham wept too.

We fell into bed early, senseless with grief.

I slept badly, waking up the next morning at five. I could not get the image of my shockingly white, dead baby son out of my mind. Everywhere I looked it was *all* I could see.

My body felt sore and ached all over. I felt like I'd been beaten up. It was difficult to sit comfortably as I was so tender. My breasts felt engorged, as if they were filling up with milk, to feed the baby who was no longer there. I could only move stiffly and was tormented with pains in my shoulders and arms, probably as a result of the anaesthetic and all the blood they had taken from me, bruising my flesh. I was able to speak now: not that I had anything to say, and my throat was still irritated, so I could only croak huskily. Emotionally, I felt destroyed.

Princess Diana's funeral was televised live on Saturday the 6th of September, and I watched it all, from beginning to end, as did most of the world. I have never cried so much in my entire life either before or since. I admired Diana for her empathy, her difference, her extraordinariness. But I also felt a bizarrely strong conviction that my poor dead baby was in that white coffin with her, borne along in state. Graham and I sobbed until we had eventually wept ourselves dry.

Days, weeks, months after that, a crying attack would frequently just happen, seemingly out of nowhere. I might not even be thinking about the baby (I tried *not* to brood) but suddenly, I would be overcome by rising tears and paroxysms of grief.

Graham, also frantic with sadness, was a great solace to me. We held each other, shaking with emotion but trying to be strong, glad of the other's support.

Every time I slept, I had such dreadful nightmares that I was frightened to fall asleep. I was always searching for something. I grew agitated, seeking feverishly, growing ever more distraught. The horror only ended when a monstrous ugly old woman, with a huge hooked nose and warts, clad in thick black cloth, would suddenly thrust into my face what I had been hunting for, what I had lost for ever: *my dead baby.* Then I woke up, sweating with terror.

People sent multi-coloured rainbow bunches of flowers and sympathy cards but, in my distraction, I hardly noticed them.

Friends and relatives came to see us: some talked about our loss; others did not. Nobody knew what to say. I grew tired of being told we'd had awful luck. I was past the disbelief stage now and was alternately depressed or angry: with God or the devil or whoever was in charge. Why had this happened to us? I asked myself, repeatedly. What had we done to deserve it? I knew it would be a very long time before Graham and I would be able to accept the enormity of the terrible loss we had endured.

My moods were unbearably volatile. Sometimes I would feel relatively normal again, even almost happy, in an unthinking way; then I would suffer another unexpected crying fit or a further slump into despair. We wanted answers to our questions immediately. *Why* had our baby died? But nobody could tell us.

I found it terrifying the way these bouts of misery just came over me. It was as if I had no control at all over my body or emotions. I was crossing a bustling main road with Graham soon after my baby's death and feeling shaky in the hot sun. I wanted to cry but felt too exposed and oppressed as there were so many people around, so I struggled to control myself. I pulled the ends of my blonde hair as hard as I could, to stop myself from breaking down.

Graham and I talked over all that had happened, constantly. Was this the end for us? We had not one frozen embryo left. Could we bear to go through the whole interminable cycle of IVF again? Should we adopt a child? Should we remain childless? The questions went continually round like a Ferris wheel, but no answers emerged.

Every time I left my house, all I seemed to see were blissfully happy pregnant women and smiling people pushing prams full of red-cheeked chubby babies. There were hundreds of them everywhere. I tried not to look. When would I be one of them? I felt that I had lost my chance forever. What made everyone else so fertile and why wasn't I? I couldn't seem to find a way of living with it at all.

Whenever I closed my eyes trying to sleep, it all ran through my mind again, like a clip of film repeating itself on into infinity. I tried to think of some pleasant episodes in my life, but I couldn't. I seemed stuck in the loop. There it was all over again: the sonographer telling me that she couldn't find the baby's heartbeat; Graham's crumpled face and shocking tears; the stunned denial I had felt. Only when I saw my dead baby lying between my legs, staring up at me with sightless eyes, not crying or breathing, had I really believed for the first time that he was truly dead. Only then, when I returned home to my baby's nursery empty-armed did it really hit me with full force: there was no baby: there was *nothing*.

Graham told me how proud he was of me, which made me feel even worse. 'You were magnificent in the hospital,' he told me. 'I don't know another person who could have coped as well as you, with all you've been through.' His praise, which was usually rare, failed to cheer me up because I felt a complete fraud. I was being so brave on the outside but inside I knew I was falling apart. I felt like an imposter in my own life.

Graham took me out on long, green forest-filled walks to make me feel better, knowing how nature soothed me. He took me to the blustery green-blue seaside, knowing how much I loved it. But I felt terribly nervous travelling in our black Fiesta and distractedly anxious when I was finally at our destination. Crowds full of strange people pulsated everywhere. Even cutting across a road became a tormenting trial for me. I was terrified of the speeding cars which all seemed to be rushing headlong right at me. I panicked in the middle of a frantic road. I desperately wanted to cry but stopped myself by sticking my fingernails into the palms of my hands: the pain emptied my flooding eyes. I now felt as if my normal protective outer layer of skin had been flayed off and I was exposed, as defenceless as the new-born baby I had tried and failed to bring into the world. Graham noticed my distress and led me off down an empty side street and talked to me, calmly, until I recovered. We discussed everything as we walked, agonising over what to do next, but we could decide nothing. We were jammed in limbo. We had to wait for the meeting with our consultant, Mr Ali, to see what he had to say about why our baby had died.

Graham went back to his work, immersing himself in it but I could not bear to go back to teaching. I stayed at home and more friends sent healing flowers, compassionate cards and heart-felt messages and it did make us feel a little better, just knowing that people cared even if we were still too distressed to read the cards or look at the flowers.

One of the white-coated hospital doctors had mentioned oh-so-casually as he was passing, that babies sometimes die in the mother's womb because there is something wrong with *her*. Why this seemingly irrelevant, throwaway remark should remain resonating in my head when so much else had passed over me was a mystery. Nevertheless, in my heightened, traumatised, emotionally anxious state, I truly believed that I was seriously *ill*. I thought I might flop over and die at any moment, probably of a coronary. I felt pressure on my racing heart and in my left arm, and my knees felt boneless and shaky. This was it! I knew I was about to collapse. I walked about the living room in a panic. I went to bed early, trying to relax but I felt stiff with tension all over. "I can't have a heart attack while I'm lying peacefully in bed," I kept telling myself, not really believing it, to calm myself down. It was an endless, torturous night. I was far too anxious to sleep.

The next day, Graham was so concerned about me that he managed to get me an emergency appointment at the doctors. I was in with the unlucky Doctor Powell for twenty minutes, crying and trying to convince him that I was about to die at that very moment! He paid attention, sympathetically, his lined face and iron-grey hair creasing together into a kind-looking whole. He didn't even listen to my beat-missing heart. He told me firmly, 'You are *not* about to drop dead. You are having panic attacks because of the trauma you have been through.' He prescribed tranquillisers and antidepressants and arranged for me to see a counsellor. He generated so much calm and reassurance that I felt better right away, just talking to him.

I started the blue and white tablets as soon as I got through my glass-fronted door, gobbling them down like Smarties.

But still, I could not sleep. I felt too exhausted and upset, as if all I could do was cry all the time. I eventually fell asleep, sobbing. I also must have been crying while I dozed because I even woke up weeping, suddenly, with a choking wail and found my cheeks and pink pillow still soaking wet. I continually expected, with cold horror, a call from the hospital telling me they'd analysed my blood, and I was terminally ill. Naturally, the phone shrilled continuously. My hand always wavered pathetically as I reached out to answer it. I was assailed with calls: Graham; my mum; my dad; my younger brother; my in-laws; my friends, all asking how I was; my headteacher, wondering when I was coming back to work; the kind woman from the bereavement office at the hospital, trying to arrange the baby's funeral.

After a week of taking the tranquillisers and antidepressants, I felt my anxiety ease a little. I stopped nibbling on my fingers all the time and thinking I might topple over at any moment, grabbing frantically at my chest. Then I felt I'd let Graham down by admitting that I couldn't cope. He told me this was nonsense. 'You're braver than anyone I've ever met,' he told me, his brown eyes melting. But I didn't feel it: I felt a complete charlatan, like a creation of frangible glass that was inundated with miniscule cracks inside that one tiny tap would shatter my whole carefully constructed exterior in an instant.

I could not get the obsessive question out of my mind: *why* had my baby died? I was tormented by guilt. What if I had, somehow, inadvertently, caused the child's death? I went back persistently over my pregnancy, thinking of everything I'd done, eaten or drunk: never anything harmful, surely? Hadn't I been really very careful?

But *something* had made my son die.

Judy, the hospital chaplain, visited us at home to discuss the funeral. I was shocked to see that she was such a tall, well-built woman when her voice on the phone was so very gentle. Comfort and reassurance flowed from her observant blue eyes. She glowed evangelically with an aura of peace and goodness. Just breathing next to her made me feel better. Nevertheless, I had dreaded her visit, fearing she might tell me bad news about my health.

'That's ridiculous,' Graham told me beforehand. 'The hospital wouldn't give a chaplain a medical job to do.' He was right. She made no mention of my being ill and I was relieved. But I was devastated at the thought of the baby's funeral. How do you say goodbye to someone who'd hardly lived? I felt my son had been a part of me and, when he died, a piece of me had perished too, a portion of my heart.

I thought it impossible even to try to think that anything could ever be the same again. Everything had changed, forever. I had become a different person. My whole viewpoint on life had altered, irrevocably. I felt so vulnerable, as if any draught of wind could just sweep me away. Now that bad luck had found me, would it keep on continually visiting me? Was I destined to be an eternal victim from now on, one for whom nothing ever went right?

I went to see a counsellor, as arranged, but the woman told me I was still "in grief" and so she could not help me yet. I did not go back. What was the point? I felt there was no reason behind anything anymore.

Chapter 15

Saying goodbye

I phoned my mum to ask if Graham could borrow Dad's black tie.

'Who's died?' she asked me, bright, curious and hard.

I just couldn't believe it.

"My *son* has died, *your grandson*," I managed to gasp, before putting the phone down and crying without stopping once again. I could not understand my mum sometimes. How could somebody who was so sensitive at times be so insensitive at others? It was like she'd immediately slipped my son into the "deny" section of her brain. She could deny he'd died by denying he'd ever existed. Deny, deny, deny. She never mentioned him once after he'd died.

My mother: the same woman who would turn on her Christmas tree lights for half-an-hour every morning and afternoon, just so the schoolchildren could see them as they went to and from school, was the woman who refused to let a Sky salesman visiting Dad use her bathroom to wash his hands, physically blocking his way, hatred and scorn on her face, just because he was black.

We decided to call him Thomas, Tom for short. I could not sleep at all the night before Tom's funeral because every time I thought about it, tears kept spilling uncontrollably down my face.

Both Graham and I were up long before eight-thirty. We were ready by nine-thirty, showered and dressed in our decent black clothes. Graham had picked up our wreath from the florist the evening before. It was beautiful, all white carnations and green foliage. We were both so tense and nervous. We strode about the house, fearful and restless. I hadn't bothered to put on any eye make-up as I knew it could not possibly stay on for long around my flooding eyes on such a tragic day. We prowled around like caged leopards until the earliest we could leave.

We were at the crematorium by ten-fifteen. We had never been there before and were agreeably surprised to see how green and peaceful it looked. Graham parked our black Fiesta, and we went to the waiting room. Nobody else was there. We carefully placed the exquisite wreath on the brown seat and resumed pacing up and down again. Judy, the saintly chaplain from the hospital arrived with her assistant, Charlotte. She had asked our permission to bring her when she'd visited us at home to discuss the arrangements. Charlotte was a chaplain-in-training and had never witnessed a funeral for such a young baby before, which was why Judy wanted her to attend. We were the only mourners as we'd asked all our families and friends not to come, having realised how upsetting it would be. We also couldn't really cope with other people at that time and just wanted to be alone with our grief.

We talked to Charlotte a little, while Judy changed into her minister's robes. Then a glistening black car drew up outside the waiting room. The chauffeur from Lloyd's Funeral Services got out and opened the back of the car and brought out our baby's coffin. At the sight of it, I started crying uncontrollably and so did Graham. I felt my shattered heart break into still tinier pieces. The coffin was shockingly beautiful, very small, only a little bigger than a shoe box. It looked like it was made of white marble, and it had ornate gold handles on the sides.

The pallbearer carried the coffin in. Graham and I had told Judy earlier that we did not want to carry it, afraid that we might drop it in our emotionally shaky state, and distressed at how light it might feel. The man put it on the raised platform under the pink-ruched curtain. Piped music played the soothing strains of *Brahms' Lullaby*.

Graham and I walked behind the coffin. We didn't know what to do but simply followed our instincts. Graham carefully placed our wreath on top of the tiny casket. It fitted perfectly, exactly the right size and looked beautifully appropriate.

Graham and I were ushered into the first row of seats by the two ministers. I went first, followed by Graham, and Charlotte sat next to him. Judy had printed twenty of the funeral service sheets as mementos for our families and she handed them to me. Graham and I had a copy each, but it wasn't much use to either of us as we were both crying so hard that we could hardly make out one word. We wept, snuffled, sobbed, held hands and dabbed tissues to our brimming eyes, all through the service.

I felt it to be a wonderfully cathartic ceremony. I was overcome by my misery in so many different places, especially on hearing the poems that Judy read which had been written by other parents who had lost babies. I responded to the real, deeply personal emotion beneath the words. I knew from the anguished feelings expressed in them that they had suffered as terribly as we had. The very worst part was the committal when the pink curtain came down and we could no longer see Tom's pathetically tiny coffin. I didn't think it possible that I could cry even harder than I was and yet I did and so did Graham. I was hardly aware that it was the end of the service and Judy was kneeling in front of us. She held our hands in hers, to comfort us. Then we were shepherded out.

At the door of the chapel, we thanked her for the ceremony. She told us she had looked at our file at the hospital and noted there were two photographs of Tom. She asked if we would like them and, my heart turning over, I said we would. She told us to tell Mr Ali at our meeting. Then Judy asked the pallbearer when we could collect our baby's ashes and he replied, "Twelve tomorrow." She hugged us goodbye, as did Charlotte and they had to return to their duties.

Graham and I couldn't bear to go home right away, so we walked around the cemetery. We were still crying. We couldn't seem to stop. We took consolation in the fact that everything looked very well-kept. We saw about twenty people dropping off white flowers and tidying graves. We noticed a special chapel which contained a book of remembrance, and we later paid for an entry in it for our Tom. (We went back on the anniversary of his birth and death to read it and there it was: "Baby Thomas Joseph Davies: always loved and remembered." It was comforting to see.)

I cried myself empty. For once in my life, I didn't care about how dreadful I looked with my puffy streaming eyes and my red swollen nose. All I felt was the overwhelming grief of my baby's death.

Eventually, we felt composed enough for Graham to drive us back. We were relieved that the funeral was over and we had laid Tom to rest officially, but I wanted his ashes very badly indeed, safely buried, as I had planned.

When we got home, Graham dug a hole at the bottom of our garden in front of the laburnum tree. I had picked this spot as it was my favourite peaceful, private place, chosen so I could always see Tom's grave from the kitchen, the living room or our bedroom window. When the laburnum blossomed, the ground was covered with a carpet of golden petals and yet more flowers streamed from its branches like brilliant yellow lanterns, lighting up the garden. I planned that this was where we would say goodbye to our son properly to be able to talk to him whenever we wanted. Then I would feel that we had laid him to rest properly, not thrown him away somewhere, like rubbish.

I had to wipe my glasses very vigorously as Graham dug, for they were all stained on the inside with the blotches of my tears.

The next day we went to collect Tom's ashes from Lloyd's Funeral Services. The casket had been wrapped in brown paper for us. I was so delighted to get it and carried it home in our black Fiesta, hugging it to my heart, with joy and peace. When I unfolded the paper, I was surprised to find a proper little box of chestnut-brown wood. It was all sealed, so that the ashes couldn't possibly fall out. There was a brass plate on the top engraved with "Baby Thomas Joseph Davies" and the date. It was perfect. I carried it reverently into our back garden. I kissed it and placed it in the black empty hole. I kissed the wooden cross we had been given by a neighbour and put that on top of the casket. Graham waited, leaning on his spade, to cover it up.

'Throw soil on,' he whispered. I picked up a little earth and smelt a faint whiff like patchouli oil. I dropped it on top of the casket. It made a final-sounding thud as it fell, scattering. 'Goodbye,' was all I could think to gasp though my heart was brimming over. Graham covered the casket with soil until the little hole had all been filled in. I cut all the flowers that were growing in my garden to put on his grave, leaving the garden barren and empty, like my womb, like my arms.

'I don't want to see any flowers anymore,' I said to Graham, firmly. I'd longed for this child so much. I didn't want him to die. Surely, he didn't want to die. But, somehow, *he died.* Nobody knew why or how.

Then I cried at my baby's final resting place, leaning my hand on the rough bark of the willow tree so I didn't fall over. But I was pleased that I'd brought him home, at last.

Slowly, gradually, we were learning to come to terms with our unspeakable loss. As Graham and I felt strong enough to return to work, we had to tell more people what had happened to us. We drew some consolation from their empathy.

I found even more comfort from bingeing on naughty food, like chocolate and ice-cream, and shopping for little luxuries with which to pamper myself. Of course, I put on weight and had no savings left but this did not matter. I needed relief and this was how I got it. Protractedly, both Graham and I began to feel a little better.

We had our long-desired-yet-dreaded meeting with Mr Ali at the local cottage hospital at the end of October. I felt nauseous journeying there, terrified of what I might hear. We waited outside his office for a good half hour and once we were called in, he explained, 'Some of Mrs. Davies's results were not on file and we had to wait for the lab to fax them through. But we have them now. You'll be glad to know that all the conclusions were negative, so that means you are fine.'

He smiled positively at me. I could hardly take it in and blinked back at him, bemused.

'There's really nothing wrong with you,' he began again, nodding his head to reassure me. 'The only positive result was for a recent virus, a very common one that you had only just contracted when the baby died.'

'I don't even remember having a cold,' I muttered.

'No. It was a virus you were probably unaware that you had. I only mention it because it was the only thing we could find. We could discover nothing wrong with the baby.' He paused, looking rather awkward and lowered his already gentle voice. 'We have two photographs of your baby on file. I believe you told Judy that you'd like to have them.' My heart jolted like it had been given an electric shock. Of course I wanted the photographs of my baby. The image that was always in my head, deeply imprinted, leapt into the forefront of my mind, once again. There he was: my boy, dead, white, his lifeless eyes staring. I shuddered yet I craved those photographs more than I'd ever wanted anything in my life. They would be all I had left of my baby.

'I would like them.'

He handed me a small, brown envelope labelled "photographs" along with the date they were taken. Then he looked up again from his notes.

'Is there anything you would like to ask?'

I took a quick breath. 'Did he suffer much... before he died?' My voice cracked. I hardly wanted to think about it, yet I had to know.

Mr Ali focussed his soft, brown gaze upon me. 'What we know of consciousness is that it's like a lightbulb, so he would only have had a very dim awareness of what was happening. I'm sure he didn't suffer.'

'Thank you.' I took a full gulp to dispel the lump constricting my throat, then thought of something else I just had to ask. 'Will it happen again?' My voice sounded high and strangely childlike, even to me.

'It is unlikely you will contract the same virus once more and, as for Down's syndrome, I think you were wise to have the triple test and hope you will again in the same situation, but you will only have the identical risk as anyone else your age.'

I felt elated. This was better than I had dared to hope. 'So, shall we get pregnant again?' came from my lips.

Mr Ali blinked and coughed, embarrassedly. 'That, of course, is a matter for you both but I see no medical reason why not.' I felt a lunatic, impulsive urge to kiss him. My anxiety had evaporated, and my heart felt light. At last we had hope again. But how could we do it? Because, naturally, it wasn't just a matter for ourselves, as for most normal, fruitful couples. Our fertility clinic would not let us have further treatment until they had all the information they wanted from the hospital, as to why

Tom had died. And how could we bear to go through all that again?

Afterwards when we returned home, I went upstairs to my bedroom, sat on my pink dressing table chair and finally looked at my treasured yet dreaded photographs of Tom. Heart thumping, I took them out of my bag, with quivering fingers and slowly opened the envelope, edging them out, millimetre by trembling millimetre. I wanted to see them, yet I was frightened. There he was, just as I always saw him in my mind, though not as dazzlingly white: his skin looked brownish, and sticky gummed. How long after he died were the photographs taken? I had no idea. Perhaps he'd been embalmed with some sort of preservative fluid while they did tests on him? But his eyes were open, and he was certainly dead.

I gazed and shuddered, yet I was glad I had the photos. I put them away carefully in my brown cabinet in my bedroom, where I kept my most precious things. Graham did not want to see the photographs, just as he had not wished to look at Tom when he was born but I had to: yet another difference between men and women, I reflected. As I put the pictures away, I cried, differently this time, tears of joy and relief that I had some solid memorial of probably the only baby I'd ever have.

The sad truth is I didn't mourn Tom properly. Nobody told me I should, or I could or how to do it. Everybody just encouraged me to forget about it and move on with my life, so I did. It was too painful to deal with my loss, so I didn't. I tried to bury my pain deep inside me but that never works. It has to come out. Time too was against us. We imagined our fertile years ebbing away and felt I had to get on and get pregnant again quickly. I regret not mourning properly now. I should have faced the pain and taken more time, but I didn't, and I paid the price later.

Slowly, gradually both Graham and I began to feel a little better. The less depressed we felt, the more we wanted to try to have another child. But it was the most difficult decision of our entire lives. We talked about it endlessly.

And eventually we decided to try again: we *had* to.

Graham phoned our hospital to inform them that we would like to return for a fourth cycle of IVF, and they were agreeable, having been satisfied by the maternity hospital that it was a random virus that had unluckily killed our Tom.

And so, Graham and I stepped back on the fertility merry-go-round. I lost the comfort-eating weight I had gained, slowly and with difficulty. Our lives once more became a cycle of hospital appointments; injections; blood tests; scans and operations. For this, our fourth cycle, I had ten eggs recovered and eight of them fertilised. Two fresh embryos were replaced but, devastatingly, they did not implant into my womb. I had to wait for two normal menstruations and then could have two frozen embryos replaced. Whenever I thought of them, a picture vaulted into my brain: a row of ice cubes containing perfect, tiny, frozen babies, their heads lowered and their legs crossed, so they looked just like Leonardo's famous drawing of a child in the uterus. I had great faith in my ice babies. All they needed, surely, was to be popped back into my womb where they belonged, and all my love and warmth would thaw them out and coax them into life.

Chapter 16

Walking with angels

In June, we'd had two frozen embryos replaced by the famous Doctor Bloom himself: one eight-cell and one six-cell. I did a pregnancy test myself on Saturday the 8th of July. I was pregnant once again and with a magical rainbow child! My ecstatic joy was this time tempered by caution and anxiety. Graham and I went, apprehensively, to our clinic for a blood test on Sunday the 12th, and when I phoned them on the Monday, they confirmed that I was indeed pregnant. During this phone call I was on a school trip, having taken my class to Tatton Park. I had to sneak away from everyone and phone them on my mobile. Annette, a nurse friend of mine told me it was the operation to remove the retained placenta from my womb after Tom died that probably helped me to conceive more than anything, as I'd had all those years of detritus cleaned from my uterus. She said she'd known several friends who'd fallen pregnant after a D & C or similar procedure. I really didn't care what had got me pregnant: I was just completely overjoyed to be so. However, our celebrations at having conceived were much more muted this time around. We'd had our hopes uplifted and then destroyed and so couldn't be as optimistic this time.

It was a long, anxious pregnancy.

Graham and I found it difficult to cope with our good news, ever aware that it could all end in disaster at any moment. Not for one single day of my interminable pregnancy did I truly relax and enjoy it or even dare to hope that everything would be fine this time. However, we progressed through the abominable morning sickness that lasted all day and night, through the nerve-racking first, second and third scans. I took the triple test again, though terrified, but it only showed a 1-in-240 chance of disability, so we declined an amniocentesis. We advanced on, worriedly, past the five month stage when Tom had died (an incredibly overwrought time) and continued.

I was petrified when I awoke on the 4th of December to find enough blood to fill a tissue. I was six months pregnant and horrified that I was losing my second precious baby. Graham and I dashed to the labour ward at the hospital and were monitored. The medical staff were worried that it was per vaginum (PV) bleeding but we were all very relieved when it turned out to be merely a rectal bleed. I had piles and one had bled! It's quite funny and embarrassing on reflection, but at the time both Graham and I were crazed with worry, as proven by medical records that stated we were both "very anxious." It was dreadful. But we survived. As the pregnancy went on I developed a strange and grim belief that either I or the baby would be sure to die. Perhaps even the both of us. It just seemed too good to be true that I should have a healthy child and survive myself, to enjoy it all.

The day before I was due in hospital to be induced, I left a farewell note for Graham in the top drawer of his bedside cabinet. "Dear Graham," I wrote. "If you are reading this then I am dead. I only hope to God that our daughter has survived. I want you to know that I love you more than you will ever know. You have been a fantastic husband to me and have nothing to blame yourself for. My death is just one of those things. If our daughter has survived, I'm sure you will take good care of her. I really think you should marry again once you find a woman who could be a good mother to our baby and a good wife to you. Try to be happy. All my love, forever, Lorna."

I had been in slow labour all day Wednesday and was already three centimetres dilated by the Thursday morning, when I was due in hospital to be induced. I'd agreed to the suggested induction because of my advanced age (I was now thirty-nine) and because of Tom's death. I was taking no chances of anything going wrong.

   We arrived at the hospital reception and were shown to our delivery room – a large, stark place, smelling of antiseptic, enlivened only by an incongruous television set, fixed high up on the wall. 'Most of the men like to watch sport while their partners are in labour,' the midwife informed us, helpfully. How very supportive, I thought, grimly. My Graham would *not* be engrossed in a football match while I was shrieking in agony, I would see to that. A young doctor started off the induction, fixing a drip of Syntocinon into a vein in the back of my left hand. At first, nothing seemed to be happening, so I could just chat to Graham and watch the sports-free television, desultorily. Then the contractions began, faintly. Having been through labour before with Tom, I knew how painful it was going to become and therefore planned to avail myself of every single painkilling drug or technique that I possibly could. Labour progressed arduously. The freckle-faced midwife reckoned I would give birth about midnight, but my body had other plans. Labour speeded along so rapidly that by the time I was in real perspiring pain, then excruciating agony and asking for an epidural, I was told, 'It's too late! You're fully dilated. It's time to push!' I had to make do with gas and air. I couldn't even tell if the gas contraption was working for all the alleviation it made to my pain: or maybe I wasn't doing it properly? It's probably not a good idea, I thought, wretchedly afterwards, to teach someone how to work a machine when they're already writhing about in torment and finding it rather difficult to concentrate.

I pushed with every atom of my hard panting being. I strained to push out the baby for two and a half hours, according to my medical records, though it felt *ten times* longer than that. I had to push down into my bottom, I was told, like I was trying to defecate an enormous pumpkin bigger than myself. The gigantic thing stuck inside me would *not* come out: it was simply too huge! It was like being constipated and striving and shoving, scarlet-faced, popping blood-vessels in my head, with a roomful of spectators watching, cheering me on to push, as if I wasn't desperate to get this thing out of me as quickly as I could, before it split me in two. But it was just TOO ENORMOUS! I felt I was being torn inside from my throat to my bottom and would crack wide open. It was horribly agonising and embarrassing. I had not one particle of dignity left. Graham was present throughout and tried his best to support me.

The midwife asked, 'Would you like to be cut a little, to get the baby's head out, as your perineum seems stiff?' I readily agreed: they could slice me from my neck to my vagina if they wanted, if this racking agony stopped. With one final God-Almighty effort, I propelled the baby's head out and with one last push, felt the rest of the baby slither out of me with a squelch like a suction pump.

My baby was born!

Graham and I both felt immediately elated with a rhapsodic, euphoric ecstasy, delirious with bliss, walking with angels!

I still noticed it was five p.m. and the signature tune of *Wheel of Fortune* was trumpeting out of the television.

The midwife wiped the cherry-red blood and white mucus off the baby, wrapped her in a blanket and gave her to me. True to the received wisdom of childbirth, I immediately forgot all the pain as I held her, and would willingly have gone through it all again, twice over, to reach the joy of that moment. 'It's a girl!' the midwife announced happily, though we already knew. I had felt in my heart I was having a girl this time, long before the eighteen-week scan confirmed it to everyone else. ('Look, a hamburger between her legs, not a sausage!' the funny sonographer had helpfully pointed out to us, when we told her we wanted to know the baby's sex. My own mother had told me as soon as I started to show that I was having a girl, 'You've put on weight all over. You do with a girl. With a boy you only put on weight at the front,' she said.)

'And she's perfect,' added the midwife, at which our emotions bubbled over even further, with relief. She added, 'How *alert* she is! Most new-borns are sleepy.' We all marvelled at our incredible Natalie, which we decided almost immediately to call her. She was looking around, taking everything in. She looked me up and down curiously as I cuddled and cooed over her, as if she was thinking, "So you're my mother." Then she stared at Graham intensely, as he spoke to her, as if thinking, "So you're my father. I've heard your voice a lot, obviously, but I did want to see what you looked like."

'She looks a lot more disappointed to see us than we are to see her,' I commented to Graham, feeling amused. It was true: the baby's face did look rather unimpressed. The midwife told us she'd slip out for a while so we could be all alone together as a family for the first time, which I thought was very sensitive of her. Graham and I just stared at Natalie and at each other with sheer exhilaration, amazed that we had done it. We had achieved our dream, against all probability and now we had a healthy baby girl. We gaped at her, astonished, dizzy, feeling drunk at our unbelievable good fortune. We were thrilled by her long, perfect body, her translucent curled-up fingers and pink shell-like nails. Her enormous blue eyes gazed at us, fixing our images in her rapidly developing brain. She even looked around the room inquiringly as if asking the great existential questions: *Where am I? What am I? What am I doing here?* She didn't cry. She was far too busy looking inquisitively around. Our jubilation boiled over. We wanted to giggle and cry at the same time. We just couldn't believe how beautiful she was or how lucky we were to have her. She was undoubtedly THE most remarkable child ever to have been born!

'It's just too good to be true,' I beamed into Graham's delighted face.

The midwife returned after ten minutes which passed like ten ecstatic seconds.

'Aren't you going to take a photo of her?' she asked, noticing our camera on the side table by the delivery bed. Graham took a photograph of Natalie at ten minutes old, lying naked on the weighing scales, crying now, for her first photo, one of so many to come.

'Seven pounds, eight ounces,' announced the midwife. 'A perfect average weight for a baby girl: and I'm sure that's the only average thing about her.' This led to more relief and happy, congratulatory glances between us, the proud new parents. 'I'll just stitch you up,' the midwife told me, in a matter-of-fact way. Because of the euphoria of Natalie's birth and the ceasing of the wrenching labour pains, I hadn't really registered the fact that I was still aware of some pain in my lower body. I didn't care. I had my exquisite healthy baby again, wrapped in her cream hospital blanket and I held her jealously close, blissfully inhaling her unique new-born scent.

The midwife took up her position at the foot of the delivery bed with all her stitching paraphernalia. She looked like a member of the Mothers' Union about to sit down at a quilting circle. The midwife stared, examined, and paused. 'You're bleeding more than you should be,' she said, in a voice she kept deliberately casual. 'I'll just get someone else to have a look.'

She left the room hurriedly, returning the next instant with the senior midwife on duty, a grey-haired woman who looked very experienced. She gawped, transfixed, at my nether regions, too.

'You've torn internally,' she said flatly. 'Don't know why. Maybe the baby's arm was up, or her elbow was sticking out? It's a big tear, from the top to the bottom of your vagina. We'll get you stitched up, but you'll probably have to go into the operating theatre for it.'

Damn, I thought. I'd known that this was all going far too well. Now I had to go into the operating theatre, the very last place I wanted to be. I wished I could stay here with my new baby and my husband and enjoy our hard-won success. Damn, damn, DAMN! Suddenly, my once-peaceful delivery room was crammed full of people. Where had they all come from? The bed I was lying on was whisked down the corridor into the operating theatre, in a riot of movement and bluish-white lights. There were even more people in there, all green-gowned and scrubbed, reeking of disinfectant. How had they all arrived so quickly? I wondered.

Graham was literally left holding the baby, totally alone. He felt shocked, he told me later. One minute the delivery room was a place of joy and calm, with just the two of us and our new baby. The next instance it was full of unfamiliar people ignoring him and the child, sweeping my bed away, running down the corridor as they pushed it into the operating theatre. He was left in complete solitude, holding our new-born Natalie, not knowing what to do. He cradled her, walking up and down, not understanding what was happening. There wasn't one person around when Graham, clasping the baby to his heart, wandered down the corridor. It seemed to him as if he'd suddenly been transported into one of those classic Westerns where the town is abruptly and magically deserted before the hero cowboy must face the massive showdown. He later told me how he wouldn't have been surprised to see tumbleweed being buffeted down the empty hospital corridor. Everyone had dashed into the operating theatre with me. What would he do if the baby cried? There was nobody around at all to ask for help. He realised there must really have been something wrong with me or they wouldn't have rushed me into the operating theatre so fast. He imagined the worst possible outcome and then tried to put it out of his mind. He found the payphones at the end of the corridor and, putting the baby back into her Perspex cot-on-wheels, phoned my mum and dad.

'Good news!' he gasped down the mouthpiece. 'Your granddaughter has been born and she's fine, she's beautiful and healthy and everything.' He waited for the yelps of delight to die down. Then he hushed his voice. He didn't want to upset them, yet he thought they should know. 'But Lorna's been taken into the operating theatre for emergency surgery.'

'We're coming right away,' answered my mum. Graham's heart soared. This was exactly what he'd hoped she'd say. Then he phoned his parents, promising to keep them informed.

Chapter 17

Dying

I lay on my delivery bed and looked around the glaringly bright operating theatre with mounting exasperation. It was like being at Euston station during rush hour. Where had even more of those green-masked and gowned strangers suddenly materialised from? The entire rest of the hospital must be completely deserted, as all the staff seemed to be in there with me. I felt incredibly annoyed. Where was my precious baby? Would Graham know what to do with a child on his own? I loved my husband, but I knew he wasn't familiar or comfortable with young babies. How would he cope?

A man approached dressed in elfish-green with a skullcap covering his hair, his mask dangling askew by the side of his face. 'I'm Doctor Harrington, your anaesthetist,' he told me. 'Would you like to be awake for your operation or would you like me to put you to sleep?'

What operation? I thought, crossly. I only needed a few stitches! Why would they want to put me to sleep, like a vet getting rid of a sick cat. How long was this going to take, anyway? I wanted to scream. I had a baby to look after now. Didn't anybody understand? Instinctively I recoiled at the thought of being put to sleep: that would take longer, surely? Time wasted putting me under and bringing me round. I would feel drowsily drugged, and maybe I'd be sick? But staying awake would mean an epidural: they were rumoured to lead to back trouble later, I had heard. What was I to decide? I had to get back to my baby and quickly, to help Graham with her.

'I'll stay awake,' I told the anaesthetist, furiously. I really felt incredibly enraged. I'd gone through the excruciating pain of natural childbirth, while being ripped apart internally with only a few whiffs of gas and air to relieve me. Yet now it was all over, they were going to give me an epidural. I could have had the bloody epidural at the start and not had to endure all that pain. Such is life, I fumed to myself: well, my life, certainly.

A nurse rolled me over onto my side and the anaesthetist gave me an injection I winced at in the base of my spine. I soon became completely numb from the waist down and they started the operation. Doctor Roberts, the registrar on duty, introduced herself as being the one who would carry it out. The operation dragged interminably on. I had no idea what was taking so long. Give me the bloody needle and I'll do the stitches myself, I wanted to shout. I'd been good at needlework and embroidery when I was at school. I longed to get back to my baby and cuddle her, holding her safe in my arms. This was absolutely the story of my life, I seethed to myself. I achieved things but was never allowed to enjoy them. Something always came along to ruin it. I'd finally attained my ambition of having a healthy baby after ten years of trying, but now I was about to *DIE* on the operating table. How bloody typical! I lay there stiffly in a frenzy of fury. I'd never been so angry in my life. If I'd died at that moment and made it to the pearly gates, I'd have given Saint Peter such a bellow of intense incandescent rage I could have cracked heaven and hell into smithereens.

It became obvious even to me, in my emotionally agitated state, that I must have torn very badly indeed and the whole assembled hospital staff could not seem to stop the bleeding. I was going to bleed to DEATH. I was in a fever of anger. The operation stretched on, endlessly.

They had placed a screen over my stomach to stop me seeing all my blood and insides spilling out, but I could easily view some horrifically gory reflections in the huge chrome steel light that hung over my middle. I tried not to look, gazing to my side instead.

After hours that felt like days of lying there, frozen, listening to anxious voices, the top consultant surgeon arrived. He swept into the operating theatre like a king on a royal progress. 'I am Mr Yakabuski,' he told me. 'There's no need to worry.' He smiled so softly, his brown eyes so benevolent, I knew I was in very bad trouble. 'I will sort everything out.' (I found out, the next day, from a chatty midwife that I was the talk of the hospital because they couldn't stop my bleeding and so had to fly in Mr Yakabuski by emergency helicopter, at great expense, from his country estate, to *save* my life!) This new consultant began to busy himself about the tail end of my body. I really didn't care about anything by then. After four hours in the operating theatre and having lost over three pints of blood, which I discovered later from my notes, my anger had finally lessened. I was relieved that they had eventually stopped poking about inside me, and that I was *not* going to die. I was, at last, ceremoniously wheeled back to my delivery room to see my poor abandoned daughter and husband.

As soon as I was pushed back in, I was surprised to see my parents there and my daughter firmly encased in my mum's doting arms. My mum looked at me and smiled when I said, 'Trust my mum to have hold of the baby.' (She told me later how shocked she was to see me: I had red and yellow blotches on my skin and was visibly exhausted. She wondered what they'd done to me.) But I lit up like the Oxford Street Christmas lights when Natalie was lowered into my eager, out-stretched arms. 'Isn't she beautiful?' I demanded of my parents. They, of course, agreed. She was even more perfect than I remembered. I sighed blissfully as I snuggled close, breathing in her sweet face and translucent skin; the flawless hands with the fingers all curled up; the pink-blushed, pearly shimmering nails. I wanted to hold her forever.

I heard my mum ask Mr Yakabuski, who'd followed my bed proudly in a victory parade with the other medical staff, how many stitches I'd had.

He tilted his head, obviously trying to count in his mind, but gave up saying, 'A lot!'

Everyone laughed, except me. It was hardly a joke. How much pain would I be in when the epidural wore off?

I wasn't even allowed to hold my treasured baby for long. My mum took Natalie again while another hovering doctor fixed a drip in the back of my left hand to rehydrate me. I couldn't walk around holding my child if she cried, for the epidural had numbed my lower body so much that I couldn't possibly move my legs.

I didn't care. We were so excited that now everyone had finally left us in peace. Graham repeated how shocked he'd been to be left alone with the baby when everyone dashed into the operating theatre. He told me how relieved he felt when my parents arrived, though still worried about me, of course. He explained how my mum and dad couldn't even get into the maternity wing, as there wasn't a soul around to let them in. For ten minutes they'd just tapped on the glass at him and their new granddaughter, until Graham figured out how to unlock the electrically coded door. My parents cooed about how delighted they were with their granddaughter and how perfect she was. I kept quiet, typically. It seemed churlish of me even to mention that I'd just nearly bled to death.

It was late evening by now and they all had to leave, shooed out by a new nurse who told them I needed my sleep. But I could not rest at all. I was left alone with my baby for the very first time, the child lying in her clear Perspex cot next to my bed. Natalie slept, flushed and innocent and I watched her. I was too excited, elated and exhilarated to sleep myself. A doctor came to fit me with a catheter to collect my urine. Other doctors checked it all through the night, making sure I wasn't still bleeding too much. Though exhausted in my body, my heart and soul wanted to sing. I lay, marvelling at how miraculous my baby was and kept discovering fresh, wonderful features to admire: her perfect upturned nose; her finely curved lips. All night I watched and listened, amazed at each new incredible breath.

The next day I was transferred onto the public ward, refusing the offer of a private room, as my friend Julie had advised me I would learn a lot on the ward.

'You need a blood transfusion of three pints,' the nurse told me. 'Unless you object.'

'Why would I object to a blood transfusion?' I asked, confused. Then I realised, 'Oh, you mean if I was a Jehovah's Witness? No, I'm not.' The blood arrived in three frozen plastic packets from the laboratory. They looked like boil-in-the-bag cod fillets, only bloated with red liquid rather than creamy-coloured sauce. It was prepared in the rather low-tech way of being stuffed into the midwife's pocket until it had thawed to body temperature.

By the evening I'd had three pints of blood transfused, one after the other, into the back of my hand and felt a lot livelier. I was also on a drip to rehydrate me. I was allowed to get out of bed for the first time, once they'd taken the icepack out of my vagina very slowly, but I still felt shaky and dizzy. I leaned on Natalie's Perspex cot as I pushed it along in front of me, to find the toilet. I couldn't fit the cot in the cubicle with me, so left my sleeping baby outside the open door so I could see her while I used the toilet. It stung, like lemon juice splashing on an open wound.

I could now get out of bed to breastfeed my baby myself, without a midwife having to hand me the child. I wasn't sure if the baby was properly latched on, but she certainly sucked away greedily.

That Friday night, my baby woke up with a high-pitched cry. It was quiet and dark. I sprang out of bed and gathered her to me. I fondled my baby's soft head to my breast and fell onto a comfortable armchair. The lighting on the ward was dimmed but I could see my child and the dusky outline of mothers asleep in their beds with babies sleeping in cots beside them. I didn't know what time it was, but it felt like the middle of the night. I didn't care. My baby gorged away on my breast, and I felt that hot flow of my milk surging outwards as the baby sucked gluttonously. I suddenly felt quite differently to how I had been feeling, like a switch inside me had been turned on. It was as if all my tiredness and confusion were swept away in a sudden surge of unexpected maternal love. This was what I had been hoping for and wanted. How things should be. My love for my child seemed to stream out of my very being. It seeped out of every pore, warming, nurturing, caring. My love wrapped itself around my child while I stroked her precious sleek head. My baby suckled yet I was the one who felt suffused with heat, full and satisfied, as if I was feeding from some mysterious healing force. I felt flooded with love. There was too much for my small body to contain. It seemed to spill out of me and spread, filling the space around me, creeping like white mist. Soon the darkened, hushed ward was completely illuminated full of my blissful exploding ecstasy. I felt completely surrounded by pulsating love, like I was back in the womb, glowing and comforted and still it swelled out to fill the hospital, then the entire town, the total extent of the country, the whole world. My love swept relentlessly on like my own universe expanding. And we were nestled at the calm, content centre of it all: me and my baby Natalie. I was so ecstatic to be a real mother at last.

But recalling my past had only taken me so far. I'd been told and read in certain books that losing a baby and having IVF were two things that were often believed to be contributing factors in developing postnatal depression. Both were not uncommon, whereas I developed postpartum psychosis which only one in a thousand women experience. Something serious had gone wrong in my past and I puzzled over it continually.

I still didn't understand why this had happened to me. Then I remembered Doctor Singh asking me about my childhood and teenage years in another key moment in psychiatric hospital. I told him, of course, still in complete denial, 'I had a happy childhood. My mum and dad and brothers loved me, and I loved them, no problems at all.'

He had the tact, grace and understanding not to laugh out loud in my sad, deluded, drugged-up face. Bless him. He smiled. He was always smiling. He was one of the most smiley people I've ever met (and it was a genuine in-the-eyes smile too, not fake). He said, oh-so-gently, as if confiding a great secret to me, 'You know, in my experience, it would be incredibly rare for someone to end up in psychiatric hospital if they'd really had a happy childhood.'

And when I said, 'I don't know why this postnatal depression has happened to me out of the blue,' again he smiled.

He almost whispered, so kindly, 'In my experience, it doesn't just happen suddenly. Most people will have had depressive and anxious episodes previously in their life.'

Of course, he was damned right. I'd had depressive and anxious episodes right from my earliest years. It was time to be brave and face the truth, to go deep into the painful murk.

Chapter 18

A bloody nuisance

In my first ever photograph I am six weeks old, a pretty double-chinned little doll in a primrose yellow dress and hand-knitted cardigan. John's hand is clenched into a fist provocatively inches from my tiny baby face. John, all of three, towers over me menacingly, as he will for the whole of his life. He is wearing a lemon short-sleeved shirt under brown-bibbed shorts, one strap of which is dislodged over his shoulder by his arm, pumped up ready to *smash* his fist into my innocent baby face. My head rests on an aquamarine frilly-edged pillow and I have turned my face away from him, eyelids lowered. I look demure and peaceful, hardly aware of my hostile would-be attacker. I will never be as relaxed again being in such proximity to him: my life will teach me this.

John stares at the camera, a look of wide icily blue-eyed, slack-jawed dumb insolence on his face, a look that I, my family, our whole neighbourhood and the police will all come to know very well indeed.

This photograph is large, eight inches by six, and is displayed on the massive, polished oak sideboard in our front dining room for the whole of my first eighteen years, a constant threatening reminder. As a child, every single time I look at it I will think the same thing but whenever I dare say the words aloud, 'Mum! He's about to punch me!' she replies, 'No, he's not,' the smoke from her cigarette creeping and spreading like Scotch mist.

Maureen, my friend of the same age who lives next door, adopted after her parents already had three girls of their own, at ten years old already boy-mad, says to me, 'You're dead lucky you! It must be great to have an older brother. He'll always look out for you and protect you and introduce you to all his good-looking mates.'

'No,' I tell her, with a sad shake of my head. 'I'm not lucky! John's not like that at all.' I like Maureen, I really do. I share many secrets with her but not these: how he attacks me any time or any way he can when our parents aren't there or aren't looking; how he shows off in front of his sniggering mates, shouting abuse at me, calling me, 'Fat bitch!' Just thinking about it makes me shrivel up inside and feel miserable, anxious and guilty. Maybe it was, truly, my fault: I had, after all, been born. It's obvious even in his three-year-old face in the photograph how much he loves being the centre of attention, the focus of the limelight in the photographer's lens: he wasn't about to let some stupid brat of a little sister take it off him or steal his mummy's love. He is first-born, the entitled male, number one and he will not give up his privileged position without a gigantic struggle that causes a tsunami of action and emotion that nearly swamps my entire life. Every time I see the photograph of that scrap of a baby I want to travel back in time and warn her, 'God help you girl because the grown-ups won't.'

Of course, there are no grown-ups in my house, but I only realise this much later.

I am sure that John, three when I was born, spent a great deal of my baby years rushing at me, sticking his face close to mine, smiling, then grimacing and terrifying me, making me wail, then he was shouted at by my parents, frightening and making me cry even more. I've witnessed toddlers do this to babies repeatedly, especially unthinking types like John, desperate for a reaction. All my earliest memories are of John hurtling around, whooshing past like the whirlwind he was. My mum would leave the house to go to the shops, five minutes away. The *second* she opened the front door John would be off and she'd be panting after him, pushing me in my push chair; glimpses of houses, people and streets would fly by my vision. Her stepmother died just before I was born but Mum often took John to see her when he was a toddler. Mum said she'd always take one look at her exhausted, puffing face and mutter, 'I'd 'ave 'im in reins!' eyes narrowed, dragging long and hard on her cadged cigarette. John did not do slow. He only had two speeds: fast and very fast. I remember him climbing up the ladder after our window cleaner. The man seemed strangely charmed. 'He's great, your John,' he would enthuse, twirling his damp rag.

'I need eyes in the back of me 'ead with this one,' Mum would complain, smoothing down her pinafore. Yet she *liked* it: tiny as I was, I could tell. 'The window cleaners got three girls,' she informed me, after he'd taken his money and gone. She flicked her orange duster casually over the dust-free dining table and said, pensively, 'No wonder he thinks John is great.' *I* didn't think John was great. I thought he was dangerous and, as Dad repeatedly called him, 'A bloody nuisance!' I puzzled over this as I sat on the floor, taking the clothes off and then putting them back on my dolls. Why would *one boy* be better than *three girls*? Surely John wasn't better than *me?* I was good, quiet, did what I was told right away, tidied up my toys: *he didn't.* He was all over the place, messy, untidy, loud and naughty. Mum never had to shout as loudly at me as she yelled at him. Dad didn't hit me half as much as he whacked John. Mum, too, smacked me much less. Yet my mum *loved* him, I could tell. He'd wink at all the girls and women who walked past. Everyone noticed him and smiled. They found him amusing. I was the still, quiet child: he was the lively, noisy one. When I think of my childhood, the picture in my mind is always the same: John in or out causing trouble; me in my bedroom, reading and writing as if my life depended on it. I was always trying to make sense of my senseless world and protect my chaotic family by holding it together from collapse. I *had* to write everything that happened down in my notebooks because my family denied everything and changed what had really happened, what I'd witnessed with my own eyes and ears, and they never listened to me.

Dad loved to talk, and I was groomed to be his receptive audience. I heard many stories about the early days. 'John would wake up and immediately wriggle out of his cot and come into our room, but you didn't. We'd go into your room and find you awake in your cot, delighted to see us and not crying at all.' My blood turned to ice when he told me this. Typical Dad, he thought this was yet another example of John being a bloody nuisance and me being the "good" quiet, obedient girl they'd trained me to become, but now I've had a baby myself, I know how odd this is. My Natalie cried as soon as she was awake (in the cot next to our double bed, not abandoned in another room with the door closed). That's how you know your baby is awake: she cries, a baby's only way of signalling, "I'm hungry/need to be changed/ need to be cuddled/ need to know I haven't been left all alone in the scary dark to face danger and die," and in the night too, of course. How very convenient for my parents and damaging for me as a developing baby. It nearly froze my blood hearing this story. Why would any baby just lie in its cot and not bawl for attention? Unless it was totally cried out, had been all alone and yelling all night long, every night and ignored with the door firmly closed. I think I'd given up calling for someone to come because nobody ever came. I feel sorry for that child, from her earliest years, crying alone, neglected, abandoned, bawling away and nobody came. No wonder my nervous system became hypervigilant and predisposed towards anxiety and depression.

John was eleven. He was supposed to be doing his maths homework. He was at the same junior school as me and was approaching the eleven-plus exam. If you passed this you got into a grammar school with the clever children and got a good job. If you didn't, you'd go to the secondary modern and get a boring job in a factory, 'With the dopes,' my Dad said. He was supposed to be helping John with his homework, but he wasn't. He was watching John with his usual hostile, glittering, pale blue eyes. John's maths book was open on the dining table, and I sneaked a covert look, over the top of the book I was pretending to read. I was horrified and amazed: it was a mess of blood-red marks. *My* maths homework book was full of ticks, "Goods," gold stars and merit marks. I was shocked by his book, but I was eight years old, so I knew enough to keep my face blank and stay out of it. I'd never seen so many angry red crosses and crossings-out before. John was wrestling with his sums and again I was surprised: they were just addition, takeaway, multiply and divide: I could do them just fine but of course, I kept quiet about this. I knew if I offered to help, Dad would say, "Oh it's Miss-Know-It-All again! Miss Bloody Smart Alec! You're too-bloody-clever-by-half you! Showing off again – just butt out!" So I did what I always did, what I'd been trained to do: kept silent, carried on reading Enid Blyton's *First Term at Malory Towers*, and tried to blend into the wallpaper for safety. John was obviously about to cop it and I'd be damned if I was getting caught in the firing-line.

John was struggling, but Dad was struggling even more to keep his temper. He had no patience and repeatedly said, 'I am in no mood!' He'd been at work all day and just wanted to sit in front of the television, watching anything and smoke his Hamlet cigars, surrounding himself with an impenetrable fug that kept his despised family away from him. 'But it's twenty-four! It's bloody *obvious!*' he shouted again, exasperatedly putting his hands through his hair so the ends stuck up. He looked like Ken Dodd, but I didn't dare draw attention to it or even smile. *Nobody* laughed at my dad or, 'You'll be laughing on the other side of your bloody face in a minute! I'll knock you into next week!' He would and he could, too. Dad's temper was about to reach critical mass and meltdown. I knew all the signs. I'd studied them for my entire life, while hiding the fact that I was doing so. I was tense all over, hardly daring to breathe when he threw his black biro down on the table so hard it bounced right off again on to the floor.

'You're a bloody DOPE, you are!' he yelled at John as he retreated out of the door to the comfort of the television in the living room. 'I don't know *why* I bother!' I didn't know why either. John was always, "A stupid dope!" and I was always, "Too-clever-by-half". We were both continually put in our no-win situation places. Neither was any good: only Dad was perfect, the undisputed Master of his own house, the King in his own castle.

It was finally safe to relax my muscles now he'd gone, okay to breathe again, so I did, one long drawn-out sigh. John moved too. He made a bolt for the front door. He always wanted to be out with his mates. I always wanted to be hiding indoors reading. We stayed out of each other's way. We never talked to each other. It would have been too dangerous to be found colluding with each other: we'd have been caught and then doubly punished. "Divide and Rule," was Dad's strategy, like all dictators the world over and it worked: nobody in our family trusted anybody else. We knew we'd all sacrifice each other in a heartbeat to save our own skins. We were all isolated, stuck in our own unique misery.

Dad never even asked about *my* homework: neither did mum. They wouldn't have helped me with my homework even if I'd asked them. A *girl's* homework or schoolwork was not important to either of them. My mum's continuous, 'Get your bloody nose outta that book!' was sometimes followed by, 'Learn to clean a bloody *toilet,* that's what you need.' They both literally thought educating girls was a waste of time: all girls were good for was marrying off to spend a lifetime banging out babies and doing all the domestic work for her husband, like we'd never moved out of the Middle Ages.

The only time John walked home with me after school was the day Mum came home from maternity hospital with Richard. John must have been *ordered* to wait for me by Dad because he would never voluntarily have done such an out-of-character thing. (I was totally baffled at school by the number of brothers and sisters who seemed to get on well with each other. I even witnessed numerous examples of the traditional protective older brother looking after his little sister. They went to and from school together and talked without violence or insults. I studied these bizarre creatures intently, trying to discover their secrets. If I'd dared to ask Dad, he would have said they were, "Just pretending, putting on an act, playing to the gallery," and I was a fool to fall for it. I'd often heard him say such things to explain away any strange behaviour he didn't understand or like. But were all these people putting on a show? Maybe it was just our family that was peculiar and odd, as it was in so many other ways. Or maybe it was my fault that John hated and wanted nothing to do with me as I was beneath contempt. Or maybe, just maybe, it was *his* problem. As with all things to do with John, I was sorry he did wait for me because he made me run all the way home. This was normal for him with hyperactivity bursting out of every pore but not for sedate, chubby little me. His frequent comments of, 'Get a bloody move on, Fatty!' were also not helpful.

We panted up to our front door like two eager puppies with our tongues lolling out. John hammered on the door and, incredibly, there was an enraged wail that could only have come from a baby. Dad let us in and, ignoring the swaddled baby with its just-discernible angry red face, we threw ourselves at Mum. I was so relieved that she was home at last after two long weeks in the nursing home when I hadn't been taken to see her at all. Thank god she was safe, also I now knew we'd get proper food for tea, not the boring cold baked beans on burnt toast which was all my dad seemed able to manage.

If I ever came across John and his gang it was never a good outcome for me: he saw to that, training me to stay away from him. I remember coming out of school once with Maureen, and John was lurking across the road with his loutish, pimply gang. He spotted me and yelled 'TITCH!' as loudly as he could. All his gang laughed uproariously, like it was the funniest joke they'd ever heard.

I was annoyed. 'The cheek of it,' I complained to her, quietly. 'Calling me titch. I'm nearly as tall as him!' I noticed the unmistakable flash of moist pity in her brown eyes.

'He didn't call you titch, he called you *bitch*,' she informed me, in a lowered, ashamed voice. It felt like a scalding slap to the face, as my burning cheeks brought stinging-hot tears welling up in my eyes. I was used to him insulting and abusing me at home when we were alone, which was bad enough, but to have to put up with it in public in front of my friends and his sniggering and guffawing acolytes was just too much. He was grooming me to keep out of his way, to make myself invisible at his approach. Not alive was how he wanted me. His hostility and aggression towards me seemed to increase in size and strength during my miserable childhood and wretched teenage years. The only thing that kept me going was the hope of escaping to university in London.

Chapter 19

Why had he attacked me?

I was going through our back garden on my way to play, when I noticed John with Colin Cassell. (*"He was snide,"* my mum said once. I wasn't sure what snide meant but I knew, even at eight, that there was something slimy about him: he always sniggered at nasty things.) He was doing it now, as a pair of John's dark school trousers were on the washing line, billowing in the wind. 'Look! Filling up with *bad air,*' he smirked to John, not me, obviously. I was eight years old and a girl: nobody took any notice of me. On this day, however, John did notice me. Normally I was beneath contempt, unworthy of his attention. I was just passing by, my eyes fixed on our back gate when, for no reason at all that I knew of John suddenly punched me in the stomach so hard that I was completely winded. I fell back on the grass: I was in agony. I could not breathe. My insides felt all mashed together like in a cement mixer and there was no oxygen in the mix. I struggled and strove to breathe, gasping, lying on the grass, writhing, in dreadful pain. John and Colin looked at me, laughed, and they both just ran off, out the garden gate into the street, giggling, leaving me all alone to face death. I really thought I was going to die, right there, thrashing about on the lawn, fighting for breath, heart racing, chest beginning to cave in. I could not understand why he'd done it. I hadn't even looked at him or Colin. I was just trying to get away from them quickly. I hadn't said one word to either of them. I was famous for my silence: it was what I was good at, what I'd been groomed and trained in by all of them: John, Dad and Mum. *WHY* had John punched me in the stomach so unexpectedly and so hard? I struggled to find the reason for my imminent death. I just flopped there, mouth open and gasping.

Why had he attacked me? It made no sense but then hardly anything in my life did. All I could think was that he was showing off to his mate. John was always doing things to impress his friends, his gang; other boys. They were all he cared about. John lived in Boy's World. This was all that seemed to matter to him, the esteem of other boys, being thought "hard" and funny. This was the code that John lived by, even at the tender age of eleven and, as usual, I was in the wrong place at the wrong time and all alone, so I was the victim: story of my early life.

My lungs felt like two crumpled-up plastic bags with the sides stuck together. I choked, caught my breath, panted and puffed. Slowly, sluggishly as I struggled to breathe, air did creep back into my collapsed lungs in little gulps and gradually the stabbing pain eased and I could gasp a little, though it hurt so much I was too frightened to inhale or exhale strongly. I managed to pant a little and got to my feet, but it really terrified me. I'd never felt like this before. I couldn't catch my breath and might die. I practically crawled slowly back into the house. Mum saw me so I told her what had happened, in short gasps.

John eventually came home later that night for his tea and Mum had a go at him, but I'm sure she didn't tell my father. She was always protecting John from Dad. She just nattered and nagged on at John and he did exactly what Dad did: ignored her completely. John could let everything Mum said just float over him like it was meant for someone else.

Not me. Every syllable she breathed was like a dagger plunged straight into my eager waiting heart and over sixty years later it's still there.

I see this incident now as part of John's training of me, to teach me to fear him, keep away, stay quiet or I'd get the same again. It was the memory of his domestic violence that kept me silent a few years later when he'd blatantly steal money out of Mum's battered old black purse that she kept in her blue shopping bag, behind the kitchen door. I *knew* Mum walked from one end of the shopping precinct to the other to get half a penny off a tin of beans because I was there trudging along with her. I knew we had very little money. John did too but he didn't care. He wanted cash: he took it. That's how he always was. He wanted anything, he just helped himself. He didn't seem to have any feelings for other people as to what they might want, what their emotions might be. It just did not register with him. The only person that ever really mattered to John was John. So, all I could do was watch him blatantly steal the money from Mum's purse and glare at him, hoping the disdain and disapproval in my eyes might *kill* him. But it didn't and I didn't tell on him because I was afraid he'd punch and wind me again. (My mum *must* have noticed money had gone from her purse, we had so little, and every penny was accounted for. She also must have known who'd taken it but, once more I'm sure she didn't tell Dad. She was always protecting John and he took full advantage of her weakness, as predators do.)

Chapter 20

Left

Mum would pelt out, slamming the door behind her. There were no encouraging words, no, "I love you" or kisses, not now, not *ever*. She'd be yelling instructions as she went. If I'd been late, the two buses I had to get home from senior school having let me down once again, she'd be screaming at me, 'Now I'll be late, you dozy little bitch and I'll be told off!' Somehow it was completely my fault that my buses had been late as though I controlled the traffic! I'd be instructed what to do: 'Set the table, tidy up, *DON'T* answer the door!' Then I'd have my three-year-old brother plonked in my arms as she flew out of the door, her eyes already far away from me, already focussed on the biscuit factory and the start of her shift. The door would crash and I'd be left all alone in the dark, cold house with a fractious toddler grizzling away. I felt so deserted and rejected. So many nights I wanted to howl along with Richard. We both felt alone and lost, and I was terrified. What would I do if a thief broke in? This was a great fear especially in the winter when it was already dark at four. I was so scared, but I had to hide it for Richard's sake. He was upset enough already. I wanted to tell my mum that I was being bullied. I'd been "Sent to Coventry" as we called it then. Nobody in my entire class was talking to me. Everybody looked the other way when they saw me.

John was fourteen. He was a precious *boy* so he could do as he liked. Sometimes he'd come home and hit me and whip me with his school tie. Nobody was there to stop him. I was a helpless fish in his barrel, and he was the one with the gun. Dad didn't get in from his overtime at work until six-thirty, so I had over two hours alone (that's if I was lucky and John didn't suddenly turn up to attack me) with Richard. I was frightened, alone, nobody to talk to or hear me cry or scream. Totally abandoned.

I was eleven years old.

My life was so utterly wretched that I just wanted to die. I had nobody to speak to, nobody to tell, nobody who could possibly understand; nobody who cared.

I resented my dad. He never allowed me to talk or listened to me or anybody else. Dad was King of his Castle. He ruled our house like an absolute monarch: Louis the Fourteenth would have been envious. 'I will be Master in my own House!' he proclaimed repeatedly, like a miner in a D. H. Lawrence story and he certainly was. You were forced to listen to him. All he wanted was a silent audience. He'd arrive home about six-thirty announcing, 'I'm tired and ready for my tea.' He'd put on the cheap, faulty pressure-cooker, to heat up the food that Mum had prepared in the day and left to be cooked. (Even my mum and dad weren't *insane* enough to make an eleven-year-old put on the pressure-cooker in case it exploded and ruined our tea: it did regularly blow up even when my parents put it on, and the food would be splattered on the kitchen ceiling where it would stick and then drop slowly off, as time went on and it dried out. How apt this was. I always thought our family was just like that pressure-cooker and often detonated, too.)

I hated my brother John. He was fourteen, a skinhead and a juvenile delinquent. He mocked, threatened, hit and terrorised me, hated me right back double, triple, quadruple. He was in trouble with the police constantly, thieving from shops, stealing money from Mum's purse, writing his nickname "Mayo," in graffiti all over our neighbourhood, having accidents, smashing windows, scooters and cars. He lived a life of unrelenting crisis, and his chaos became ours too.

I often have nightmares and hellish flashbacks to that wretched time when I was only eleven and left alone in the house to look after Richard. They're always the same: I'm frightened. It's dark. Fears torment me. What if Richard had an accident? What would I do? What if some other disaster occurred? Richard couldn't do anything as he was just a toddler of three. What if Dad didn't come home from his overtime? His bus might break down. (Later, when he got an old banger of a car, I worried that he might have a car crash!) I wouldn't know. Nobody had mobile phones or computers in 1970. We didn't even have a landline telephone. I had absolutely no way of contacting anyone or them reaching me. I was completely on my own. What if my mum didn't come back tonight? What would I do? My parents were always angry and arguing. What if they ran away? What if they killed each other when they were rowing? I was too young for all of this. Mum and Dad seemed to think I was grown-up, but I wasn't. I only felt about seven. I was panicky. I was terrified of the dark and it was pitch-black. I feared ghosts by now. I thought our house was haunted. Mrs. Bamber who lived in our house before us had died there, so she possessed it and might come back. I feared burglars breaking in too. I was petrified of all sorts of things: everything! It was not fair. Nobody else had to do this. Not John. He was fourteen and a boy, so he did whatever he liked. I was terrified. I wanted my mum or dad to come home. I tried not to let Richard know I was afraid. He was only three. I had to put on a happy face. I was always hearing strange noises upstairs. Every so often I'd hear a dreadful knocking, 'BANG bang bang!' Once Dad was home and heard it too. He shouted, 'It's just an airlock in the pipes. Only a baby would fear that!' But it was so loud, like a monster was trapped in there and trying to break out, using a hammer to knock the water pipes. I had to put on a brave face. What would I do if thieves broke in, like on *Z-Cars*, with stockings over their heads, their noses flattened and their faces distorted, carrying crowbars! I'd be so terror-stricken, I'd just freeze, and I'd probably die of fright!

Mum shouted at me again before she left for work, but it wasn't my fault I was late home from school. My bus just didn't come. I waited and waited, feeling more and more nervous. I was dripping with anxious sweat. I wanted to shout at the bus driver, "You're late! My mum is waiting for me. I must get home quickly so she can go to work. Now she'll yell at me again!" But of course, I said nothing. I had to swallow down all my anger. I *knew* Mum would be extremely anxious and upset. She looked at me with real hate in her narrowed, hard eyes when she screamed at me. It made me shrivel up inside. Why was *everything* my responsibility? I didn't ask for any of this and I was far too young anyway. Why did I get blamed for everything that went wrong? It wasn't my fault. I hoped John didn't come home before Dad. I dreaded this most of all, feeling sick with fear. He hit me whenever he caught me alone. I screamed at him. I shook with anger all over my body. I bellowed it out. I hated him. I would murder him if I could because I knew he wanted to kill me: he always had. But he was a lot bigger than me. He was fourteen, a big, lumpish brute, a shaven-headed skinhead. He was *scary*. He was like Mum; I never knew what he'd do or say next. He never did what he was told: he didn't have to. 'I do what I like, me,' he'd say, always bragging about it. He terrorised me, chased me about the house. He loved to hear me scream. He sniggered, made fun of me, wound me up, loved scaring me; enjoyed tormenting me. He stole money from Mum's old battered black purse. Mum needed every penny, I knew. We had hardly any money. Yet he took it and he looked at me, daring me to tell. He knew I wouldn't. He knew I was too scared of him. I was frozen, couldn't do anything. I was helpless. I was hopeless.

And so I *ate*. It calmed me down. I lost myself in food. I escaped into a good book. I tried not to think, not to feel. Dad always said, 'Nobody *cares* what you think, Lorna. Nobody wants to know how you feel, so button it!' So I did. I didn't speak or feel. I made myself numb as if I were dead, like I didn't even *exist*.

When I got home, I wanted to complain and cry to my mum about the other girls being horrible to me, but she just shouted at me for being late which again felt totally unjust. The unfairness of it stung my eyes and I cried when she went but I had to hide it from Richard. He was only three and I didn't want to disturb him. I didn't want to upset anyone.

When John terrorised me and whipped me with his school tie it drove me so mad with anger that I stood on the landing, gripped the banister and *roared* with rage. Nobody was there to hear. John had gone out to cause trouble with his mates again. Richard was watching children's television. Even if anyone had heard they wouldn't have paid me any attention: nobody did, but bellowing with fury made me feel better, letting all that pent-up frustration out. I felt furiously angry but then I felt overwhelmingly sad. I had nobody to talk to. Not one soul understood me. Nobody knew or cared what I was going through. I felt so isolated, so depressed. I think Mum needed to see me as stronger than I was, maybe to ease any guilt she may have felt at leaving and using me, but I knew I wasn't strong, and I was too immature for all this responsibility. It was too much for me. What if Richard fell and banged his head and it bled? He had bashed his head twice, both on the metal fireguard and on the tiles around the fireplace. Luckily both times were on a Saturday, so Mum was there to hold a wet flannel to his head until the bump stopped swelling, but it scared me…

but then *everything* frightened me. If he had another accident, a worse one when I was on my own, what would I do? We didn't even have a telephone so I couldn't call an ambulance.

My stammer got worse and worse, and I flushed bright red. I stared at the ground as I walked. 'Stand up bloody straight!' My mum would yell at me. 'What is wrong with you, walking all hunched over?!' I couldn't even ask for what I wanted in the local chicken shop. I felt like the loneliest, most isolated child in the whole wide world. I felt like I walked around with the outer layer of my skin flayed off. I was so painfully vulnerable and exposed. I was bullied at school *and* at home. I had no respite. I kept it all in, but I felt I would simply burst or go mad some day.

I craved affection from anybody, but especially from my mum. I wanted her love, desperately but all she gave was food to fill my bottomless emptiness. I ate and ate and ate but it was never enough.

Chapter 21

Domestic abuse

I could never sleep when I was a child. I would wriggle about and sigh all night long. I always had a lot going on in my mind so was often over stimulated and could not relax or clear my mind enough to rest. The second reason was that I had such terrible and recurrent nightmares that I was afraid to doze off.

I still have trouble sleeping now. I regularly have flashbacks and anxiety dreams about the abuse I suffered at John's hands. In my bad dreams someone is always chasing me. I flee, *terrified.* I think I've escaped into a room, and I slam the door and put my back to it but the monster pushes at the door and shoves against it, ramming it open. It forces me to be propelled forward even though I have my back pressed to it, am leaning all my weight upon it and am thrusting back on it with my full strength, feet planted on the floor. But still the door is pushed and forced open and shoved, thuds and bangs as it opens a crack and is forced closed again by me. I'm screaming, petrified but the monster is determined to break into the room I'm in, trying to get to me and hurt me badly. I often wake up suddenly, heart hammering, sweating, gasping and afraid.

Of course, this happened to me time and again as a teenager. I'd be chased around the house by John, and I'd end up leaning against the living room door, my back pressed to it, and he would be using all his weight to force his way in and batter Richard and me. I'd scream hysterically as the door jerked and shuddered and I forced it back and closed. I had to protect Richard: this was my given role by my parents. I didn't ask for it or volunteer. I had no voice, no say in it at all.

John subjected me to this domestic abuse (I didn't know what it was, naturally, as a child) terrorising me and it went on for years: my entire childhood and teenage years. I told Mum and Dad, but they didn't allow it to inconvenience them: they did nothing except yell at John even more, but he just shrugged it off. No wonder I was so traumatised, so damaged, so afraid of everything. The worst thing is it does stay with you for life. Every stress in my life triggers memories of comparable terrible things that happened in the past with similar bad people, so that I feel it's happening all over again with double force. Then I just want to blot out all the pain by any means possible.

I bolted my bedroom door from the inside every single night. I didn't have a proper lock on my door, of course. Even our toilet didn't have a lock on it because my Dad was, "A lazy, obstinate sod," to quote my mum, so I improvised. Luckily, I had the metal part left on the wall side of what must have once been a proper lock or bolt. I discovered that if I jammed a broken wooden coat hanger through the fixed diagonal handle on the door, it would slot into the metal part and effectively bolt the door rigidly shut. It would have taken quite some force to break into my bedroom and, at least, I would have heard the racket and had some warning.

I know I did this all the time I lived in my parents' house, from childhood onwards. Mum would regularly shriek at me, 'Why do you do it? What if there's a fire? You'll never get out. You'll be burnt to a bloody crisp!' But obviously other things worried me more than a fire. I continued to bolt my door every single night. What was I frightened of? *EVERYTHING!* For as long as I can remember I've been afraid, anxious and mistrustful. My earliest memories are all pervaded and stamped by fear. As a tiny child I was terrified of the dark, the unknown and monsters. As I got older, I learnt to be afraid of ghosts and of boys and men and their menace, of the threat of burglars, thieves and rapists. I was taught, *groomed* to be frightened of my father, my older brother and my mum, their sudden inexplicable mood swings and even more swift random violence. Our front door was flimsy, old and could not be locked at night, so I feared bloodthirsty, destructive men breaking in. My childhood home was not *safe* either inside or out, so as often as I could I barricaded myself in my bedroom, the only space I felt safe, the only place I felt I could breathe easily, the only room where I could relax and be myself and do as I wished and write and read, my sanctuary and haven.

It was John I was *most* afraid of and his malign attempts to have control over me. It was all about power. He loved to scare me and make me frightened of him.

He *did* and I *was*.

This is my childhood: me, still, small, silent, sensitive, eyes fixed on *Her,* Mum the Giantess, hoping, wishing, praying, silently pleading with her, with my sad kicked-puppy eyes, "Please, please love me. You *must* love me. I'll do anything for you, anything: all I ask is that you love me." But she didn't, her eyes always darting elsewhere, distracted, on her boys: John's trouble and Richard's problems, arguing with Dad, her other younger siblings ("our kids") obsessed with cleaning, her work and colleagues at the biscuit factory... anything except me, who desperately needed her attention but didn't get it. This withholding of love, making me work for it and earn it, when her boys got it unconditionally, I thought, fulsomely, unquestioningly, is beyond cruel. Making me, a child of *eleven* do her work for her, look after her three-year-old so she could do what she wanted... and still I was just used, abused, shouted at, manipulated, tortured by her love for others, never me.

My nanna told me she was, 'Only allowed to eat the scraps of food left after I'd waited on my father and four brothers, and they'd eaten their fill.' I *knew* what this felt like. I had only the scraps of affection left off my mum after she'd actively loved everyone else first: John, Richard, Dad, her brothers, her sisters, her dad, her work colleagues, John's many girlfriends... I felt *starved* for practically my whole early life both literally and emotionally. I still eat emotionally, trying to fill the yawning black hole inside me that should have been filled with my mum and dad's love but wasn't.

I was fifteen. It was well over forty years ago, yet I can still see it before my eyes. Certain scenes or images remain playing on a loop in my mind and I see and hear it all over again. Arguing: raised voices. I was writing an essay in the front room, my fountain pen filled with my distinctive turquoise ink. More arguing, louder voices, the usual. I'd programmed myself to ignore the customary chaotic background noise in our volatile house, then much louder arguing. Higher raised voices: serious. I rushed into the back room and saw Mum *pinned up* against the wall by John. She was a tiny woman, barely five-foot tall and slightly built. He was a broad fat lout of five-foot eight, eighteen years old, every *day* of them trouble. His meaty hands were on her slight shoulders.

'Don't go out, John. You know you always get into bother,' she was insisting.

'I'm going out!' he was asserting.

'You *can't* go out!' she persisted.

'I'M GOING OUT!' He jerked her shoulders and slammed her head hard against the wall that connected to the front room. Her head thudded backwards. She cried. I'd never seen my mum cry before, except over Christmas dinner. I'd seen her angry, most of the time, fuming away as she dusted and cleaned, seething away like a volcano about to blow its top. Anger was her default mode. She was and remained the angriest person I've ever known. She always shimmered and pulsated with fury: a woman never happy: a woman who rarely got her own way. But these were not tears of frustration: she was used to being frustrated. These were tears of pain and fear. I felt horrified as I stood there, helplessly. My big brute of a brother was *attacking* my mum, as he hit me when nobody else was around to stop him. I had to do something to stop him but what? My fountain pen was still in my hand. If it had been a knife, I would have plunged it into his heart or anywhere else on his body that I could reach. If it had been a gun, I'd have blown his bloody head off. But all I had was my ink pen, so I shook it in his direction violently spattering him and the wall with turquoise ink. I felt so furious, so full of incandescent rage I could have cracked all the planets circling around the universe with my bare hands. I was screaming at him, hysterically, 'GET OFF HER! LEAVE HER ALONE!' (No swear words: I didn't swear in front of my mum, or she'd go mad.) Incredibly he did take his hands off her, pushed me out of the way and stalked off, face gloomy as night. The front door slammed. He'd gone. Thank god!

My poor Mum was shaking all over, upset and traumatised. I tried to comfort her, tried to calm us both down. I was shaking all over too, with fury and adrenalin. I was too angry to feel fear. I hated him so much, wanted to kill him so intensely, there was no room for any other emotion. Yet I couldn't offload all I was feeling. I had to swallow it back down, absorb it; suck it all up, as usual. I had to calm down and look after Mum: it was my designated job. Only then did I notice little seven-year-old Richard standing in the room, looking frightened and upset, which made me feel even more furious with John. Mum wiped her face dry with a tissue, tried to hide her pain, her disappointment with her favourite child. She stiffened herself together, buried her distress, didn't want to talk about it; didn't join in when I called him names. Deny, deny, deny. It was how she lived, how she coped. Deny her favoured, entitled oldest son was a violent, out-of-control, manipulative, selfish *swine,* who didn't care who he hurt or what he did as long as he could go out, cause trouble and have a laugh with his mates. It was all he wanted to do so it was all he did. Nobody could stop John doing exactly what he wanted: not then, not now, not ever, *never.* His wishes were all that mattered. There was no thought, no concern for other people, how they might feel, what they might want. He was Lord of his Universe: he could do whatever he wished and get away with it.

My mum tried to brush away her anguish. I put on the kettle and made her a cup of tea, a feeble attempt to cheer her up. Mum's Law: at times of stress, make a cup of tea. At times of celebration, make a cup of tea. It was all the same. And smoke cigarettes too, a fistful, an armful: it was her way of coping. It made her ill, triggered stomach ulcers, angina, rheumatoid arthritis, strokes: it would kill her in the end: *John's fault.*

We never spoke of this incident again.

We never speak of anything, *ever.*

She didn't tell my dad (out at table tennis, as usual, as it was a Friday night.) Deny, deny, deny. "We are a happy family. We all love each other." This was what she told the world, all the Other People. It was a barefaced *lie.*

I didn't tell my dad. She told me not to. We are a dysfunctional family. We don't love each other. This is the *truth.* And we never talk about it or anything else, ever.

Mum nagged Dad solidly for two weeks to redecorate the living room. He refused, of course, as usual. So, she got *me* to do it. That Friday night when he was out at table tennis, even Richard helped, as we stripped all the wallpaper off and painted the living room walls pink. We tore off the turquoise ink splatter on the wallpaper that must have *agonised* her every time she saw it. Now it was painted over, gone, *vanished,* never to be seen or spoken of again. If only I could wipe it from my mind so easily.

I was still wracked with anger and horror. I felt helpless, powerless and worthless. *Nothing changed.* I felt nothing would ever change. I was a horrible, emotional mess and feared I would be for the rest of my life. And John would carry on doing exactly as he wanted. And my mum would deny, deny, deny and smoke, smoke, smoke and drink endless cups of tea. All frozen in time like dead flies in amber.

Dad repeated, 'Nobody wants to know what you think, Lorna. Nobody cares what you feel, so button it!' Nobody listened. I had nothing to say: best to keep quiet. We don't talk about that. We didn't talk about *anything.* I still had no feelings in my body below my head: in my mind, a maelstrom of thoughts, feelings, actions, impulses. As I walked grudgingly to school, I told myself over and over, "*Nobody* can look into your head and see what's going on in there." This comforted me and kept me going. I was free in my mind. I was safe. My thoughts and feelings were my own. They were true and real. Nobody could deny them because I wouldn't tell anybody. I would keep it all in, to myself and nobody need ever know. I would write it all down when I got home, safe in my room, hiding; door bolted. Below my neck I still felt nothing. I was tense, numb, stiff as a coffin lid, rigid. I could stick needles in my legs, arms, breasts and still feel nothing. It was like I'd had my throat cut. I had *no body.* I was *nobody.*

I could not cry. I do not cry. For days, weeks, months, years, I cannot cry. I will not cry. I don't even know *how* to cry. I sit and I think, and I simply cannot cry.

I was afraid that if I started, I wouldn't be able to stop. I was like a figure made of sugar and if I cried, I'd be dissolved in the torrent of tears. All that was me would be gone. I don't cry because *I can take it.* I would not cry because I was strong and I would not give in to tears, weakness, messiness. This was not me. I was in control. I would not cry.

I was tense, inflexible. My head ached. My neck was stiff. I could not sleep. Again, downstairs, raised voices, shouts, yells, arguing. I could not sleep. I must make things right. I must be good. Our family was like a rickety shell of a building and if I put any pressure on it at all, the whole edifice would collapse, down, down, down into a pile of firewood. I must not wreck our boat, or we would capsize and be shipwrecked off the Skeleton Coast like my granddad was. I must be *perfect.* I must be *invisible.* I must not make any difficulties. Only John was allowed to make trouble, to be a problem. I was good. I would heal my sick family with my goodness. I would sacrifice my lifeblood to cure my dying, diseased family and I would resurrect it from the dead. We *will* be a happy family. We will all love each other. We will have no secrets. We will all talk about anything and not have to watch our mouths, not have to tiptoe on eggshells, not have to stutter and stammer and deny, deny, deny.

I would be good in school. I would be top of my class. I would get the best exam results. I would be head girl. I would win a scholarship to a private school. I would be the first in our family to go to university. I would be the first in our family to get a good professional job. I would rescue our family name from the mud. You could rely on me. I was responsible. I was sensible. I was conscientious, it said so on all my school reports. I was a good girl, invisible, silent; no trouble at all.

I had a deep black hole inside me. No matter what I put in it, it didn't get filled. I shovelled in mountains of food, cake, chocolate, sweets, crisps, pounds, stones, tons of it. But I still felt hungry all the time, ravenous, starving.

I did not talk. Mouths were for eating not talking; I'd been taught by my mum. I carried on eating. I scoffed whole kitchens full of food. But it didn't fill the empty black hole within. I was still hungry all the time.

Sometimes the deep black hole that lay within me bled like a womb and ached like a wound, when I was attacked physically, verbally and emotionally. I nursed it as best I could. I rocked backwards and forwards on my chair, soothing it. I hid in my room. Mum's family came to visit but I pretended I wasn't in. It was easy. I was very quiet, like a tiny, little mouse. I kept still, barricaded in my room. I read and wrote as if my life depended on it. It *did.* I wrote down the *truth,* so when it was denied by Mum, by Dad, by John, at least I would *know.*

One day John went too far and had his head shaved: now he was the complete skinhead. His mate Pete was the first to get his head shaved and now John had copied him in his brainless, sheep-like way. Dad went completely berserk when he saw him. I was surprised the bomb squad didn't come round to investigate the cataclysmic explosion. Dad shouted, swore and threatened. The whole neighbourhood shook.

'You're not allowed out for a whole two weeks to give your hair time to grow a bit!' Dad decreed. This was a terrible punishment for John, who only ever wanted to go out with his gang but even worse for the rest of us because John, who was too idiotic to pass even one single O-level, had a Masters' degree in the dark art of Making a Bloody Nuisance of Himself. Wherever he was, whatever you were doing, he would make so much noise, create so much mess, start so much trouble that you would want him away from you, at any price. I used to (silently) wish him dead in various horrible ways and pray to God that there wasn't a hell, so I'd never have to come across him again. I seethed inwardly; then held my breath when he loitered near me, wondering what fresh torment I was in for. John treated me like the dirt beneath his feet, but I consoled myself with the thought that I was good compared to him. He got away with all his dreadful behaviour, of course. He always escaped any punishment off Mum. Oh, she'd warn him and shout at him, but nobody ever took any notice of Mum's nattering and nagging, except *me*.

I resented my dad, too, both for how nastily he treated me himself and because I viewed him through my mum's jaundiced, prejudiced eyes. She regularly poisoned my mind against him, like some women do when they are divorced from their husband, but Mum managed to do it while we all lived in the same house! My Dad sometimes acted as my champion, but I felt he was just asserting his will against Mum and against John, as usual, so I couldn't thank him for it. Anyway, I didn't want his love, his attention. I wanted my *mum's,* but it was always taken, like the engaged sign on a public toilet, firmly in place. Her heart was always filled with overwhelming love for somebody else: John.

Finally, he went completely too far and even Mum couldn't get him off with it. My parents had paid into an insurance policy for me since I was a baby (as they did for both my brothers, too.) They paid in a few coppers a week and when I was eighteen it paid out: EIGHTEEN POUNDS! It doesn't sound a lot: it wasn't but this was 1977 and it was the most money I'd ever had in my existence. I spent the lot on something I'd longed for all my teenage life: my own stereo radio cassette player! It was *the best thing* I'd ever had in my entire life. I had it for four blissful weeks when I could lay in bed and listen to the charts and Radio Luxembourg on it. Then John spotted it and grabbed it off me one evening when our parents were both at work. He refused to give it back. He always just helped himself to anything he wanted, so he didn't see why my one and only prized possession in the world should be any different.

John then went out to see his mates. Dad got in from work and found me in devastated tears, so I told him what had happened. He searched John's bedroom and found my radio cassette stashed away. He gave it back to me. He put the silver chain in its bolt on the front door and watched television while waiting for John to return.

Mum came home from work. John returned home later, having been out causing mayhem with his gang. When he tried to get in through the chained door, Dad heard and was waiting for him. John seemed surprised he couldn't get in with his key. He pushed at the door and the chain. Dad growled at him. I'd never heard such venom and testosterone in his shockingly new deep low voice, even more frightening for being so controlled. I'd heard Dad lose his temper a hundred times and go completely berserk and it was scary, but this was worse: there was something *animalistic* about it, something primeval.

'Go away,' he rumbled. It seemed to come from deep in his bowels. 'You don't live here anymore.' John tried to force the door, but Dad repelled and grappled with it, the old wood of the door groaning and shuddering. I was afraid it would splinter and break. I could hardly breathe. But John, unable to get in, was forced to go away again.

Mum was hysterical in the kitchen, 'Oh GOD! My poor boy! Where will he go?' She was weeping and wailing, much more concerned for John than for Dad or me, ignoring John's crime, as usual. I was hiding at the top of the stairs terrified they might murder each other, or John might kill Dad and then me, but Dad prevailed, thank god. It was good of Dad to take a stand and throw John out for stealing my cassette player, but I do think, as always, Dad acted in his own best interests first. John was getting increasingly out of hand and Dad seemed very glad of this excuse to get rid of him once and for all. He also correctly surmised, in his Machiavellian way, that my daft Mum would blame me for it, as much as she held Dad responsible: no change there. So he grabbed this opportunity with both strong hands. Also, John was a big lout of twenty-one and a trained chef. It was only his doting mummy who worried that he'd be unable to survive.

I still feel guilty as I recount these horrific events that happened to me, as if I'm breaking the family's code of silence. "We don't talk about such things. If we don't mention them, they never happened." I feel I'm not only talking about the elephant in the room, but I'm also riding about my parents' house standing on its back, like I'm a circus acrobat, screaming, "Look! This is the reality, the truth!" I'm not so much as alluding to the skeletons in my family's closet, I've taken all the skeletons out of the closet and I'm dancing around the room with them, screaming, "Look! This is it; how it really was!" I feel most guilty about my mum, of course. All her life she lived by her own code of mafia-like silence, repeating, 'This stays in the family!' Deny, deny, deny. She always maintained, 'John's not a bad lad really. He's just misunderstood. Yes, he got into a bit of trouble, but it was never his fault. It was other people who led him into bad ways.' Rubbish. John enjoyed the excitement of crime and never gave it up.

My parents, especially my mum who I felt closest to, were always *altering* my reality. They were constantly denying my actuality and invalidating my feelings about it.

My teenage life was hell and there wasn't one thing I could do about it. Something happens to children when they have no respite, no relief from their torment. They turn in on themselves. When I left primary school, I was a happy, popular (voted head girl by the other girls), outgoing, friendly girl. At eighteen, when I left Redcoats,

I was introverted, withdrawn, overweight, stammering and painfully shy. I could only relax on my own because I couldn't believe or rely on anybody. If a child can't trust her own family, her own parents, to put her best interests first, who can she trust? *Nobody.*

It's intensely painful to remember all of this, so many horrible memories deeply stored away and repressed, things I couldn't possibly have coped with at the time. They would literally have blown my mind, so I suppressed them, "helped" by a family who also deliberately tried to forget it all. "Deny it ever happened," was the family motto, closely followed by, "Pretend we were all happy, that we all loved each other," conveniently ignoring the fact that John was a juvenile delinquent skinhead criminal.

It's still a lot of pain and misery to deal with but I keep reminding myself that this all happened in the past. It can't hurt me now. I'm safe and away from it and it doesn't matter if my family denied it ever happened, as was their usual way. I know it did and that's what matters. I'm not the "mad" one anymore. I can face the truth and the reality, and they can't. I'm not the deluded one, lying to myself. I'm healthy and strong because I can accept the horror of my childhood and teenage years, and they can't. Truth will out and I'll be the better and healthier for facing it.

My mum used me as her waste bin where she dumped all her toxic trash and then stuck a lid over it firmly so that it didn't get out. Only years later did I explode, and she claimed to be puzzled as to why this happened. It had nothing to do with her, she'd been a perfect parent, as had my dad, they were very keen to tell my psychiatrist. I was never allowed to offload on to her. On one occasion I was so desperate I told her a little of my misery at being bullied at school. The next day Dad *went* for me, furiously and viciously, 'DON'T go telling your mother things that will upset her!' he thundered in my face as he pinned me to the wall in the hall. She'd obviously repeated everything I'd said to him the second she could: no wonder I couldn't trust her. Yet Dad upset her every single day, and the boys did too. They were allowed to tell her "bad" things; then she immediately dumped all her worries about them on to me. I felt so anguished and as time went on, I felt worse and there was nobody I could tell, nothing I could do, just suffer, keep it in and feel even more agonised.

I was terribly bullied at Redcoats, of course. Brought up as I had been, I practically had a "Gift to Bullies," neon sign over my head. I'd been groomed at home in not standing up for myself, never allowed to be assertive. I'd had all my self-esteem and confidence beaten, terrorised, belittled and humiliated out of me long since. I was like a fleeced sheep tossed into a pit of wolves. It was painful and isolating but I stuck it out and told nobody: no-one listened to me anyway. It was horrible but being bullied at school was not as bad as being bullied 24/7 at home: at least I could get away from school. But I could never get away from Mum, Dad and John's bullying, that was constant, and it was living in that continuously stressful environment for years on end, with no respite that most harmed me and adversely affected the rest of my life, until I learnt how to cope with it.

John was undoubtedly a catastrophe, born barely six months after they'd been forced to marry. Richard was a surprise (born over eight years after me. Mum had thought her family complete with a boy and a girl. She was thirty-six. 'I'm far too old for all this,' I heard her complain to June next door while pegging out the washing. 'I thought I was finished with all this nappies and bottles stuff! I'm making the beds at nine o'clock at night!')

What was I? An accident? A mistake? Almost certainly. Contraception didn't seem to be a strong point with either of my parents.

Mum loved John best of all, I thought, right up until the day he died and the day she died and beyond, more than she loved me, who always took care of her, like a substitute mother should. He was the child of her heart, and I could never compete with that, no matter how well I looked after her and did all her work for her. I loved *her* but she loved *him*: you don't expect to enter the eternal triangle from the moment you're born!

I made three solemn vows to myself. One: I will *never* turn into my mother. Two: I will *never* marry a man like my father. Three: If I have a child, I will *never* bring them up as I'd been raised. If I could achieve these three things, I'd feel I'd lived a good life. This was what I aimed for.

The tragedy at the core of my mum's failure of a life happened in 1937 when her mother died: this was at the root of why she didn't know how to be a mother.

The tragedy, the poison, at the source of my father's failure of a life was Uncle Andrew. His malign influence was the reason he didn't want to be a husband or father.

Mum did the physical part of motherhood well. We always had an immaculately clean house, lots of food, freshly washed and ironed clothes but the emotional nurturing part of mothering she knew nothing about. Deprived of it herself, she was hopeless at it.

Dad did not want to be a husband. He considered he was "caught" by Mum getting pregnant with John and he took his resentment out on her, on all of us, for the entirety of his life. He also didn't want to be a father. He repeatedly said we were all just drains on his resources, and he took his bitterness out on all his children for his whole life.

Chapter 22

A life worth living

I learnt so much from my therapy, often from the most painful things. How devastating it was when Doctor Singh asked me once, 'Whose voice is saying these things: "The baby must die," and "You must die." Is it a voice you recognise?' And he smiled so kindly, so reasonably.

'It's *my* voice!' I gasped, amazed. I really was shocked. How could I be saying these terrible things? Yet it was after that realisation (I can pinpoint it to that exact moment) that I really started to get better.

One of the most stupid and pointless ways human beings can spend their time on earth is arguing with yourself in your own head but this is what it's like to be "mad." Even when on the outside I looked blank, like *nothing* was going on, this was always running on: arguments raging, anxiety churning, like volcanoes constantly erupting in my mind, tornadoes swirling and tsunamis flowing, my thoughts constantly at war: no stillness to be had at all in a mind in conflict with itself. And you'll do anything to stop it and find peace, even the supposed calm of death and self-annihilation.

Soon after I gave birth to Natalie, I felt like I was at my lowest ever ebb (physically, mentally and emotionally) at the very bottom of a steep valley, then down the slope of the mountain came, like a steam train, faster and faster, all the accumulated baggage of my thirty-nine years and it smashed right into me: and that was my postpartum psychosis. It knocked me out then flattened me. All the incidents and issues of my life that had gone beforehand that I hadn't dealt with (Tom's death; the reality of having a live baby and looking after it; my pre-natal depression; my anxiety; my emotional volatility; the abuse I'd suffered in childhood from Mum, Dad and John, physical, verbal, mental, emotional and financial; all the things I hadn't been allowed to say; all the questions I hadn't been allowed to ask; all the things I hadn't *dared* to face or even think about, emotions bottled up, not processed, all denied) SMACKED into me with tremendous force. I had an awful reckoning, its moment of revenge on me, like bullies waiting and then getting at you when you're down and at your lowest point. It smashed into me all at once, loaded carriage after loaded carriage after loaded carriage until I broke into a million fragments.

The most important thing Doctor Singh ever said to me was at one of our last interviews. He asked me what I was doing, and I told him.

'That's good,' he enthused. 'You're getting on with your life. You know…' he confided, softly, 'you may have thought you did but nobody really wants to kill themselves and die. What people really want is a life that's worth living.'

I absorbed these wise words into my very soul. He was exactly right: that's what I wanted, what we all want: *a life worth living.* But how to get one, that was the problem. What made my life worth living and how could I get more of it? I puzzled over this for years.

My abusive parents brought up John to be bad and me to be mad. They damaged me, made me frightened and passive so other predators could abuse me too; and they did. Crucially, at the lowest point of my life, when I was at my most vulnerable, when I'd finally managed to have a child of my own, that's when the years of abuse and damage really flattened me, like a ton weight.

But I found resilience within myself. I got better. And I didn't bring up my daughter as I was brought up. The poisonous legacy of abuse can be broken.

I've come to terms with how I was brought up and healed myself in the process. I have learnt, accepted and forgiven; and found peace, serenity and contentment. I have forgiven them all, even John. I saw how viciously Dad battered John and bullied him and how mistakenly Mum protected and colluded with him. They made him what he was in the same way they made me what I am and Richard what he is. I can also forgive Mum and Dad. They in turn were made as they were by their parents and families and the sexist patriarchal culture that damages us all.

This has been the story of my long journey towards empowerment after being totally disempowered by all around me as a child and teenager. It has taken me most of my life, a long, difficult, traumatic journey and many hard lessons learnt. I had to stop letting my abusive family keep dragging me back so they could use and abuse me again. I kept on trying to make them love me and be the kind, caring people I wanted them to be. When I discovered I couldn't change them because they didn't want to alter their behaviour, I knew I had to stop. I realised I wasn't that needy child anymore. I didn't need their "love" or their "approval" or their "attention." They were the ones with the problem, not me. I also realised that my happiness was as important as anyone else's: that other people had continually treated me as a doormat because I'd given up my power to them, so I had to stop giving my power away and take it back where it had been taken from me. I distanced myself from these hurtful people as much as I could and cut ties with them. I know now: I am in charge of my life, not them. I've learnt to be assertive and stand up for myself. Now I am happy and empowered.

I was walking at the local country park with Graham. We passed the play area by the lake, and I noticed the mother first, in a bright red coat, sat on a picnic bench. She was dragging on a cigarette and staring at the lake, her children ignored. Then I noticed the boy with a mop of blonde hair. He looked about five. He was advancing on the other child, probably his sister. I could only see her back, blonde hair cascading down her pink coat, strapped into a pushchair. She was so small that she looked about two. The boy came close up to her, smiling at first, then he contorted his face into a grimace, pulling his face into scary shapes and he hissed at her through clenched teeth, 'Die! Die! Die!' The girl emitted terrified wails and roused the mother, who nattered at the boy, 'Leave her alone, David! Stop making her cry. How many times do I have to tell you…'

We walked on past, but I felt shaky. This had been a wake-up call to me.

'John used to do that to me.'

'Yeah. Sibling rivalry. Kids are horrible to each other,' said Graham casually.

But I felt tense with shock. This was the source of my visual and aural hallucinations. This was why the smiling babies on the congratulatory cards had transformed into scary faces, coming out at me. This was what John had probably said to me, "You must die! The baby must die!" in his childish, jealous rages. This was what had traumatised me and been reawakened in me when I was ill and exhausted after Natalie was born. This was *why* I'd developed postpartum psychosis, long-buried horrible memories of trauma. I walked on mechanically, my mind revolving.

My early abuse led *directly* to my postpartum psychosis, coupled with my failure to mourn Tom's death properly, and being left alone to cry all night as a tiny baby. Being left with a helpless baby triggered all my awful childhood memories of being left alone aged eleven looking after three-year-old Richard while fourteen-year-old John chased us around the house to batter and terrorise us at will. I soldiered on by myself after my baby was born, never asking for help because in my abusive family I never got any help. I was raised to put up and shut up, so this is what I did, and it led directly to my postpartum psychosis. My family didn't help because they never did, all too self-absorbed. I was there to help them, never the other way around, they thought and, of course, a difficult baby needs more than one person looking after it. As we all know, it takes a village to raise a child. I thought I was a failure as a mother and so I wanted to die. I couldn't see how I could cope, how I could do it. The psychiatric hospital and staff, especially my motherly nurse Enid showed me. I learnt. I recovered, slowly, and with setbacks (still attracting abusers) until I learnt how to say "no," and stand up to bullies but I continued to learn, getting better and better at it. I have changed so much. I was a pushover for predators and let others walk all over me, the "nice" girl, raised never to say no to anyone but now I say no a lot. I'm assertive and much happier because of it.

I distinctly remember Janice, one of my favourite nurses saying to me, 'Come this summer, I'll see you proudly pushing your pram down the high street, and I'll know you're fine again.' I thought this outrageous comment was impossibly audacious. Though this was exactly what *did* happen, one gloriously sunny afternoon, that wonderful summer and we both laughed out loud together, when we spotted each other, at her prophecy come true. And I realised I was more than fine, I was actually *happy*. I also saw her two years later in Asda, when I was holding my daughter's hand and laughing with her, every inch the devoted mother. I said to Janice, 'Why didn't you say hello?'

'We're not supposed to,' she told me, 'In case it identifies someone as having been in psychiatric hospital.' I'd been so busy just living I'd hardly thought about the hospital for ages. Why was it considered so shameful to have something go wrong with your mind? If I'd had a broken leg nobody would have given me anything except sympathy but because my mind had not been working properly, I should be stigmatised! It didn't seem right. Natalie was now three and was the absolute centre of my existence and I could scarcely believe there was a time when this had not been so. She was a real personality now with her own delightful ways of responding to life and every day with her was a new adventure. Every single day our bond had grown stronger and now it was unbreakable. I knew we had overcome our difficult start to her life and had made a good, fulfilling life for ourselves with Graham. As I smiled at her, and she giggled up at me, her too-fine skin flushing pink, her eyes laughing, I realised I wouldn't have changed anything for the whole world. She had given me back my life and it was now a life that was well worth living.

Milton Keynes UK
Ingram Content Group UK Ltd.
UKHW010712050224
437294UK00018B/702